PRAI

Gaddis tells her story with precise and beautiful language. But most profoundly, she chooses to tell that story through a collection of flickering, shimmering moments of loss and healing, profound sadness and intense joy. *Mosaic* is a remarkable yet relatable story of what can be learned from life's harshest moments. Gaddis's writing makes space for all of it to shine through.

—Pepper Stetler, author of *A Measure of Intelligence: One Mother's Reckoning with the IQ Test*

Mosaic made me want to curl up with a cup of tea and my cat, a bouquet of flowers and my journal nearby, which is another way of saying that Laura Gaddis's memoir opened my heart in unexpected ways to love and grief and joy. I found myself delighted with the book's inventive shape. To give loss its proper place in our lives does require new ways of telling our stories, and Gaddis shows us how to do this. Be prepared: you will be changed by this brave and tender memoir.

—Daisy Hernández, *A Cup of Water Under My Bed: A Memoir*

Laura Gaddis went through it. She gets it. And she writes about it powerfully in *Mosaic*, her memoir of pregnancy, loss, hope, love, resilience, and joy.

—Ann Hood, New York Times Bestselling author *Comfort* and *Fly Girl: A Memoir*

Mosaic is a moving exploration of love, loss, and the delicate, yet unbreakable threads--or welds--that hold us to the ones we've lost and the ones who are present. This book illuminates the journey of living with grief while finding a way to keep hope alive. It is the story of a mother navigating the spaces between what could have been and what is. Gorgeous. Deeply moving. Incredibly felt. A story of learning to live with grief amidst love. Of what could have been and what is.

A beautiful book of motherhood, of loss, and how and why we risk heartbreak again and again. Though our personal stories are different, as a mother of a stillborn daughter, I could relate and felt seen and comforted by the pages.

—TaraShea Nesbit, author of *The Wives of Los Alamos* and *Beheld*

MOSAIC

A Memoir by Laura Gaddis

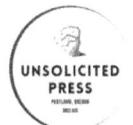

Mosaic
Copyright© 2025 Laura Gaddis
All Rights Reserved
Published by Unsolicited Press
Printed in the United States of America.
Updated Second Edition: August 2024

All rights reserved. Printed in the United States of America. No part of this book may be used or reproduced in any manner whatsoever without written permission except in the case of brief quotations embodied in critical articles or reviews.

Attention schools and businesses: for discounted copies on large orders, please contact the publisher directly.

For information contact:
Unsolicited Press
Portland, Oregon
www.unsolicitedpress.com
orders@unsolicitedpress.com
619-354-8005

Cover Designer: Kathryn Gerhardt

ISBN-13: 978-1-956692-91-4

For Jason, Evelyn, Sophia, and my angels

I wouldn't change a thing.

TABLE OF CONTENTS

PART 1: BROKEN PIECES

Terms I Need to Understand	1
Four Times Around	4
Making It	18
Support Group	23
Generalized Anxiety Disorder (GAD)	36
Criteria I Need to Meet to Self-Diagnose (Part 1 of 4)	40
The Troll in the Laundry Room	47
The Odds	49
Things They Don't Teach You	58
The Question of Religion	62
Diary	66
Criteria I Need to Meet to Self-Diagnose GAD (Part 2 of 4)	68
Walking the River of Grief	70

PART 2: TILING PIECES

Terms I Need to Understand	83
Ice Cream	86
13-Week Appointment	90
Fusion	98
Fusion (According to My Mother)	113
All the Things	119
Well-Meaning People	125
So Cliché	130
What I Needed to Hear	131
Message Board	132
Dr. Walsh Saved My Sanity (And Proved What I Thought Was Right)	139

PART 3: ART IN PIECES

Terms I Need to Understand	151
I Knew	156
Hoosier	158

Seeing Evelyn	162
Journey	169
Alarms	173
Moving Baby	175
NIC2	178
Going Home	180
Pumping	183
Candles	186
Criteria I Need to Meet to Self-Diagnose (Part 3 of 4)	189
Therapy	192
The Yellow Braces	207
Erasure	211
[Arthrogryposis] On the Playground	221
Diary Remix	224
Criteria I Need to Meet to Manage My GAD (Part 4 of 4)	226
Things I...	230
You Are My Sunshine	232
Cry and MTF On	248

PART 4
Things I Have Learned	257

MOSAIC

1: Broken Pieces

TERMS I NEED TO UNDERSTAND[1]

Rainbow Baby: a term for a child born to a couple who have previously lost a child due to miscarriage, stillbirth, or death during infancy.[2]

Recurrent Pregnancy Loss (aka Recurrent miscarriage): two or more consecutive pregnancy losses. In many cases the cause of RPL is unknown. After three or more losses, the American Society of Reproductive Medicine recommends a thorough evaluation. About 1% of couples trying to have children are affected by recurrent miscarriage.

---

[1] When I first became pregnant, I assumed it would go as planned. Just as I had seen others do as they journeyed from the first trimester, to second, to third, to baby. At the time, I wanted to better understand what the doctors suggested was happening, what tests and medicines I should have, and what new groups and categories of people I now fell into. Once I began my search for understanding, I couldn't stop. I Googled every new term, every idea, every message board, pregnancy website, and medical site I could think of: Thebump.com, Wikipedia, WebMD. I used new terms in my blog posts at sophiastory.com. I didn't dare write down a record of it all though--I mentally kept track--memory is faulty, hopeful, less consistent, less final. The rest I left to the growing electronic medical record that followed me.

[2] When I lost Sophia during my first pregnancy, I read a blog post that talked about a woman's 'rainbow baby': the light after the storm. I believed my second pregnancy would be my rainbow baby. Then my third. By the fourth pregnancy, I began to lose hope that this was a real thing.

I was sitting on the edge of the exam table, my shirt pulled back down to cover my belly. I remember looking at my knees. I had nothing else to look at. The ultrasound screen was black. The lights, blindingly white. My hands, oddly still. I remember sighing. Sighing as if I expected this news. Sighing as if I felt destined to hear her words. Sighing because of another failure. Sighing because my breath had nowhere else to go.

Dr. Akiya had told me, Insurance companies will often only cover the costs of genetic testing after the third loss because that's when they consider the losses a 'condition'.

Maternal Fetal Medicine (aka MFM, aka perinatology): a branch of medicine that focuses on managing health concerns of the mother and fetus prior to, during, and shortly after pregnancy. They act both as a consultant during lower-risk pregnancies and as the primary obstetrician in especially high-risk pregnancies. After birth, they may work closely with pediatricians or neonatologists. For the mother, perinatologists assist with pre-existing health concerns, as well as complications caused by pregnancy.[3]

Missed Miscarriage (aka delayed miscarriage, silent miscarriage, missed abortion): when the embryo or fetus has died, but a miscarriage has not yet occurred.

---

[3] I didn't know at the time that once you enter a relationship with MFM, it's for life. A blemish on your record. A relationship I didn't know I needed, didn't want to need. It was a relationship that became toxic for my mental health. But nobody told me that my anxiety disorder would spike because of false claims, overabundance of tests and appointments, and rude bedside manner. No one told me that the doctors who were supposed to know more than anyone else still could not save my babies. And that they would do so with a cold touch, a dry eye, and a smileless face. And yet, without them, my babies and I would have been more at risk.

When I went in to have a checkup during week nine of my second pregnancy, I was optimistic. I had heard the heartbeat the week before, I had no bleeding, and my gut told me this time 'was it.'

But the doppler machine only picked up one heartbeat.

I chose to wait for the baby to come out naturally. I waited four full weeks as I went on a pre-planned weekend getaway to a bed and breakfast, came home late that Sunday afternoon and grocery shopped at Pick n' Save. I sat at my work desk the next morning and administered psychological exams to others' children, came home each evening (that week and the next, and the next, and the next) and watched the local news—followed by the nightly national news—and Dateline's murder mysteries on Fridays. At week four, I wondered if it was ever going to happen. Afterward, I told myself if I ever found myself in this position again, I would not wait for the baby to come on its own. I would not do what felt the most natural—let my body expel what wasn't good for me—if that meant I walked around for a month with a dead fetus inside.

FOUR TIMES AROUND

No matter how healthy I tried to be, no matter how many foods I expelled from my diet (wine, margaritas, coffee, tea, lattes, lunch meat, tuna subs from Jimmy Johns), it wasn't healthy enough. It wasn't enough to keep my babies growing. It wasn't enough to keep their hearts beating and safely in my womb.

I was determined to make one of my pregnancies different. Perhaps number four would be it.

I estimated my new doctor was about my height, 5'6". I was thirty-three and I presumed she was around thirty-eight years old. That age difference somehow made me feel better about her as my new doctor. I didn't want someone younger, even though I didn't really have a good reason to not trust a young doctor. She had no gray hairs peeking through her brown locks and her skin was smooth and clear. She was a bit overweight, but that had become a normal risk in all of our lives since McDonald's appeared on every street corner and the line of coffeehouses in every city's downtown had bestsellers with names such as "caramel macchiato" and "mocha fill-in-the-blank." Sugar and fat and a hell of a lot of calories in every meal has made even those who should be the healthiest—those who specialized in health as a living—some of the least healthy.

She wasn't the reason I lost my three previous pregnancies. She didn't even know about them yet. Though, I'm sure my file followed me from Wisconsin, the last place of residence where we thought we'd have a child and then didn't.

She was a stranger, the third OB/GYN I'd had in five years, and the one who I had to place my full trust in as I entered this fourth pregnancy. She was very much like the others, but somehow it was also a fresh start.

"Hi, Laura," Dr. Wagner said as she peeked through the light that shined through the cracked door. She had knocked twice but I was too nervous to respond.

"I'm Dr. Wagner, how are you?"

"Doing okay," I said. Her hand, as I shook it, pressed cold skin to my clammy palm.

"Good, good. Let's see what we have going on." She rolled her stool up to the computer station. The clicking keys were grating. "Congratulations on your pregnancy. How far along do you think you are?"

"I'm not sure, but maybe like eight weeks?"

"I see." Her eyes rarely left the screen. "Looks like you have quite the history here with pregnancy."

"Um, yeah. I do."

"Tell me about it."

How do I tell a stranger about the blood-filled days at work and the soaked sheets at night? The trip to the ER? The ultrasounds that always indicated when our babies were disfigured, not growing, or deceased? Waiting for the second pregnancy—which had been declared a "missed miscarriage"—to naturally terminate as my husband and I went on a pre-planned weekend getaway to a bed and breakfast. The inn served wine and cheese every afternoon. I wondered if I was harming the dead fetus inside of me. I drank anyway.

I would have to tell her how we found out, the day before my birthday, that my third baby had no heartbeat, and how I was scheduled to have the Cytotec inserted on my birthday. My doctor at the time said, *If I had realized it was your birthday, I would have told you to wait until tomorrow to do this.* I had wondered why she thought that would have improved my birthday.

    I knew Dr. Wagner could read that all in my file. What it didn't reveal was the guilt I felt drinking the wine, because what if my baby really did still have a heartbeat? Or what it felt like to wait over four weeks for my body to dispense of dead tissue while I went on about life. Each day checking for blood. Each day awaiting the cramps. Each day expecting my baby to come out onto the floor of Target, or the toilet at work, or my bed sheets in the middle of the night. Or the conflicted feelings I had while awaiting the birth of my first child when we didn't even know if she would be stillborn. We did know that her limbs bent abnormally. Her chin receded too much. Her growth had stunted so much she was two weeks behind the curve. It didn't document the questions that plagued my mandated bedrest during the days leading up to her birth: Should I look at her? Hold her? Give her a name? What was the best worst-case-scenario: seeing her alive or dead? The file didn't quote me when I told Jason after each loss, "never again. I'm not doing this again."

    Dr. Wagner's chattiness gave the appearance of a take-charge attitude. Maybe it was how she asserted her confidence. Maybe she used it as a coping mechanism. I imagined that when your first conversation with someone is about the three miscarriages they have had, anxieties must be present.

    "I had a woman once who bled a puddle all over the floor," Dr. Wagner said.

    My eyes widened. I was embarrassed, more for that other woman whose personal story of bloodshed was just shared with me than for myself for having to hear it.

    "Oh, gosh," I said.

    Dr. Wagner pointed to the floor, marking an oval that spanned from the insole of one of her feet to the other.

...

By the fourth pregnancy my anxiety spiked on the ride over to Dr. Wagner's office. I left a little early, and even though the drive was only a few minutes from the neuropsychology clinic where I worked, it felt like the three-thousand mile journey my husband, Jason, and I had taken when we moved from the West coast to the East, driving up Route 1 along the Pacific, crossing over the Rocky Mountains from Spokane through Idaho and on to Missoula, Montana, and farther through the Black Hills of South Dakota, the flat plains of Minnesota, across the Mississippi River into Wisconsin, and finally south through Illinois, Indiana, Ohio, West Virginia, and exiting Virginia. In reality, my drive to the doctor's office consisted of: out of the clinic parking lot, onto the road, east a few miles, and park again.

    The drive should have been restful, meditative, had I been able to focus on the other cars, the browned leaves rustling in piles on the street, the school buses making their rounds to drop off children at their homes. I should have breathed in the crisp North Carolina air and felt the February chill freeze the insides of my nostrils. Had it not been for the anxiety, I could have focused on the music playing, the sun's early setting on the late afternoon horizon, or the engine rumble of my eleven-year-old Toyota Matrix. Yet, my focus was on the tight grip I had on the steering wheel. Beneath my gloves were white knuckles and sore tendons. I could feel the fleshy pulsing of my heart as the chambers constricted and retracted, pushing the blood through the veins and arteries, to and from itself. It reminded me that a heart is always beating, even when I can't feel it. I liked it better when I couldn't feel it.

    I sucked at the air as my lungs refused to allow much past my upper chest. Each breath was shallow and unfulfilling. My stomach knotted and I had to pee. I knew from before that having to pee (a lot) is just one of those shitty pregnancy things. But this time it was different. Or maybe it was just enhanced. When fight-or-flight took over my body and my sympathetic nervous system revved, my bladder always screamed (even if there was nothing to scream about). It was as if my entire body wanted to rid itself of a toxin.

…

For this appointment Jason couldn't leave work when I did. I made it for as late in the day as possible, as I also didn't want to leave work suspiciously early and have to tell everyone where I was going. In a small office with only two psychologists, one other psychometrist, and a secretary, nothing went unnoticed. I had worked there four months, and only Karen (one of the psychologists), who had become a quick friend, knew my history. I remembered the first loss, announcing my pregnancy to my former coworkers, to a chorus of happy tears, only to have to re-announce the loss to sorrowful ones. I couldn't bear to do that again.

Jason was the person I counted on to make me do the things I didn't think I could do. When I had to white-knuckle my way through a first day at a new job or go to a social gathering where new people would expect to talk to me, or for me to talk to them, he was my tree to lean on. When the winds picked up to a hardy breeze, I could cling to his lowest branches. When the breeze changed to a gust, I could wrap my arms around his trunk, fingernails clawing at the crevices in the bark. His roots dug deep and kept him still. He kept me grounded. His branches swayed with life, with the ups and downs. Even when he was worried or scared, he remained stable. I was never sure how he did it. Or if he did it. I wondered how much his own roots were searching for something even deeper to wrap around. Was there something beyond the dirt, the layers of the earth? If his roots let go, and the dirt that kept him planted gave loose, I would have lost the only way I knew how to cope. Dirt flying in my face, loose pebbles pelting my skin, tumble-to-the-ground-together kind of cope. Or maybe he felt as I did, clinging to me in some way to give him enough power to give back what he could.

...

"We have some big news," I said to my parents, five years earlier when we still lived in Wisconsin. The small ranch Jason and I bought was only twenty minutes from the home where I spent the latter half of my childhood. We stood in my parent's kitchen. I suspected they knew I was pregnant, even though I was only eight weeks along, even though I wasn't showing yet, even though we had barely spoken the words to anyone. What else would a young couple mean when they say they have 'big news'? Jason and I waited until my grandmother, who lived upstairs in my parents' house, was ready. We sat around her living room: Grandma in her tan recliner, Mom and Dad on the floral couch, me on the half-wooden chair. Jason stood by my side. My dad had just gotten a new digital recording device. It was aimed at me.

"We're having a baby," I said. I wasn't sure if my voice wavered at that moment. It felt like it wavered. I couldn't hear myself. I felt the reverberations through my skull as the words bounced. I felt joy. Or just nerves.

"How wonderful!" my mom said. "Maybe you'll have twins!"

Oh god, I hope not! I thought.

To my mother, I supposed, having two meant I would get the job done in one pregnancy. She had one sister. My dad had one brother. They had had two children: my sister and me. I wondered if she thought I could be the overachiever of the family and complete the pattern in one turn. I didn't want that responsibility. The idea of growing one human being was bizarre and unnerving enough—I wasn't sure I could handle two.

What are the odds of having twins anyway? I thought.

"I don't know about that!" I said.

Everyone laughed. Was the laughter because my joke was funny or because of the giddiness a pregnancy brings? This would be the first grandchild for my parents. It would be the first great-grandchild for my grandmother. It was a moment where those who were not pregnant celebrated the excitement of a new member of the family and where my smiles came from a place of uneasiness. I was, after all, the one carrying this child. It was my body that was about to expand, grow a second human—a parasite, really—and expel it out of a much too small hole when the baby itself could no longer fit in my torso.

I laughed, too.

Jason and I returned home later that evening. I was quiet on the ride.

"You okay, babe?" Jason asked. We hadn't even made it to the freeway entrance ramp a few miles up the road.

"Yeah, I guess so. I'm tired." I said. After a pause I added, "and worried."

"What about?"

"What if I can't do this, Shnookie?" 'Shnookie' was a nickname I made up for him shortly after we graduated from college and moved to our first cheap, rat-infested apartment on the eastern edge of Baltimore. 'Honey' was what my mom called my dad, so I couldn't use that. 'Jason' was so formal, yet still usable at times. But when I wanted to be extra cute, or look for extra sympathy, I needed something else. Snookie was the girl on Jersey Shore. So, Jason became my Shnookie.

"You can. I'll be with you. You'll be fine." He took my left hand with his right. His other hand steadied the steering wheel. "We got this."

"I know. I mean, I know I have to do this—I don't have much choice at this point."

I didn't realize then, at that moment in the car, on the ride home from what was my parents' and my grandmother's happiest moment in a long time, that in only a few weeks I'd have to deliver the news, over the phone, that something was wrong with the baby.

I didn't expect that this would be the first and last time we'd make that announcement and have it immortalized on a recording.

...

I called my mom after the terrible doctor's appointment. I wanted to hear a voice that would take away the fear that blossomed from figuring out how to proceed with a pregnancy that was nonviable. I wanted to hear a voice that mimicked mine, with the intensity of a strawberry so ripe it was on the verge of rotting. I wanted to feel like someone understood what it was like to be me, what it was like to feel the anxiety from something so out of my control. I wanted to hear my mom's voice.

I tried to steady my words, but knowing what I had to say next, I couldn't even hear myself speak.

"Mom?"

"Hi, Laura," she said. "How did your appointment go?"

She knew I had a level two ultrasound—a test I learned only the day before was a more intense, hour-long imaging of the baby, measuring every possible measurable thing.

"Not good, Mom," was all I could say.

"Oh, Laura. What happened?"

I sat back on our green corduroy couch. The oversized throw pillows that Jason's aunt had bought us to go with the couch when we first moved in together did nothing to comfort me now.

"She's not going to make it, Mom…."
"What? Why did they say that?"

"Laura?"

The silence was pocked with my attempts at swallowing sobs.

"She, she… she has some abnormalities they called it. They did an amniocentesis to see if there are any chromosomal problems, but we won't get those results for a while. The first set of results come in two days, then we have to wait two more weeks for the rest."

"Okay, so we don't have all the information yet," my mom said.

I felt like a child again, sitting on her lap as I cried about anything that made me fearful. Anything that felt out-of-control. Her tone taking hold of my worries and wrangling them with her practical ways. While at times I found this infuriating—times when all I wanted was to be heard for the sadness or the disappointment that simmered within—it was what I needed right now. It saved me from drowning in the death. From the fear of giving birth (a thought I hadn't had time to think about until that afternoon). From the notion that I would be a mother of a dead baby soon. Maybe tomorrow. Next week. Or not until I'm nine months along and she has perished in my womb. My mother's tone took me away from having these thoughts and dammed the sobs that threatened to drop tears on my blue jeans.

"No, but they were pretty definite that she won't live. They said it was a 'nonviable pregnancy' and her condition was likely 'not compatible' with life."

"I know this is hard, Laura, but let's wait until we know all we can."

My fingers, one at a time—my index, middle, ring, pinky—traced the outline of my thumb nail.

"Okay?" she said.

"Yeah, Mom."

The doctor had said the amnio may give us some idea of what went wrong so we can better help with future pregnancies. But I didn't tell this part to my mom. I wanted to feel the comfort I used to get from being wrapped in my mom's crocheted Afghan, one that had jagged lines of alternating brown, orange, and green, and smelled of yarn mixed with my mother's Jergens lotion.

Julie, the genetic counselor, wouldn't have spent an hour showing us handouts on genetic conditions and what normal chromosomes should look like if there was a chance that it would be okay. She wouldn't have talked about the twenty-five percent odds of this being a recessive genetic condition and that our chance of a future pregnancy being normal was seventy-five percent. I wouldn't have just endured an hour-long ultrasound with the technician pushing the wand so firmly into my belly, trying so hard to make my baby with low fetal movement move that I felt as if knives were sliding into my ovaries. The ultrasound technician at yesterday's routine appointment wouldn't have told Jason and me that she had to leave for just a moment and turned the monitor away from our view. She wouldn't have returned with my doctor. They wouldn't have talked in hushed voices pointing to the screen still hidden. The doctor wouldn't have demonstrated with her own hands, bending them so far, her index and middle fingers touched the inside of her wrists, insisting that our daughter's hand did this permanently. She wouldn't have continued on by telling us how our daughter's knees were not moving and were, in fact, bent at sideways angles crossing each other in an odd manner.

None of this led to a good test result.

...

Later that same year, at six or seven weeks along, we told my parents about a second pregnancy, and only three weeks after, revealed to them that the baby's heart had stopped for inexplicable reasons. The oversized gray sweatshirt I wore that day—the one that had "Middlebury" stretched across the chest in bold blue letters (the ink slightly crackled from many washings), the one that my parents brought back for me when they took off for Vermont one fall as I continued going to my high school classes—did little to hide my sadness. My mom and dad stood at the end of the kitchen counter, just as they had when we had told them we had a big announcement before. Apparently, this was the spot for big announcements, good or bad.

My mom hugged me from the side. I couldn't stop holding onto the counter. My tears became hers.

…

By the third pregnancy, I learned caution. I learned to temper all excitement.

"So, we want to be cautious about announcing this, but we are pregnant again. Only about six weeks, so still very early," I told my parents, this time over the phone. "We aren't telling too many people. Not until we know this one will go better."

"Okay, Laura," my mom had said. "We are hoping for the best this time."

We had all learned to temper excitement. And it was worth it when at twelve weeks, this baby's heart stopped, too.

…

I was now listening intently to Dr. Wagner say the patient who had bled all over the exam room floor went on to have a healthy baby. I couldn't help but think of my other babies. Her horrific tale gave me hope. I wasn't the only one who bled during pregnancy. I wasn't the only one who tried again and again. I wasn't the only one who had to take extra measures, extra pills, have extra ultrasounds and blood tests. I imagined I wasn't the only one who lost my excitement back at pregnancy number one.

After three losses, I had learned to hold in the news that once had been so joyous. Even during the first pregnancy, when I was twenty-nine, scared, and unsure that what I was doing was the right thing, a spark was there. Even the smallest of flames could ignite a maternal instinct unknown to me before. When we had told my parents back then, I found joy buried amongst the muck of worries (am I ready for this? Do I know how to be a mom? Are our finances stable? Is it enough to support a baby who needs diapers, formula, food, wipes, daycare, and onesies, shirts, pants, and pajamas that continually increase in size? Plus, who knows what else)?

This fourth time around, I told my parents about my pregnancy just as I had for the second and third ones. But this time it felt like I was announcing my fourth miscarriage before I even lost the baby. I called my parents, who now lived eight-hundred-and-four miles from our new residence in North Carolina. It was my first pregnancy on southern soil, so perhaps that would make all the difference. Something—just one thing—different might make this time work.

Dr. Wagner continued talking about the woman who bled profusely. "She just had to be monitored closely. Oh, and she took progesterone. Have you taken that before? With your other pregnancies?" Dr. Wagner's fingers furiously clicked the keys. Her eyes skimmed each page quickly, looking for all the answers.

"Um, no? I don't think so."

"It can be given in several ways, you'd likely remember it. It can be a shot, or a suppository, or just a pill you take. Any of those sound familiar?"

"No, I don't think so." I repeated.

"Well, let's try it," she said.

I felt a twinge of excitement to be taking these pills. Yet I thought, nothing else worked, so why would this?

"Good, good." Dr. Wagner patted my knee before she turned around to add to my chart.

I smiled weakly. At least, I figured, it couldn't hurt. This time just might be different.

...

This new identity as a mother, a parent, one who is responsible for another being, didn't automatically come with a flair for intuition. I had always been someone who made decisions based on what I felt was right. An empath of sorts, or so my sister, Sarah, would say. I felt energy; I felt which people carried positive energy and who carried negative. I felt in my gut what was right and what was wrong. Separating what I thought about a situation and what I felt about it was easy.

When I chose what college to go to, University of Wisconsin-Madison wasn't the one I wanted (I had fallen in love with University of Illinois, Urbana-Champaign), but something in me told me Madison was where I should be. So, I went. When I had to decide where to study abroad, I pondered several choices. Madrid called to me, more so than the Galapagos Islands off Ecuador (but that also sounded awesome). Only later would I learn that it led me to my husband, Jason. My intuition led me to move to new cities, new states, new realms of my not-so-comfort-zone. It led me to my first baby, and then the second, and the third—to all the piles of blood and ashes—to this pregnancy, and now to Dr. Wagner.

...

There was a knock at the door. The receptionist opened it a crack and said, "Jason's here." The undergraduate math course he taught at Wake Forest University was finally over for the day. It was time to start his job that required him to take in all the details Dr. Wagner gave. He was the one who listened with reason and logic. The one who tempered my fear and eased my worry that we'd lose another baby, even if he harbored the same feelings. The one who pointed out long ago that our chances of having a baby without the recessive gene was seventy-five percent, so the odds were in our favor. He was the one who could look when I had to turn away—from the pictures on the monitors, the baby in my arms, the dead child on the scale, the ashes in a box.

He took a seat next to me. He searched for my hand.

"Hi, Jason. I'm Dr. Wagner. I see you guys have had a long history here, so we're going to do our best to make this one work. I have discussed with Laura starting her on progesterone. But she can fill you in. We're going to do all we can."

He nodded. I smiled at him until he seemed to relax.

"We have a game plan, guys," Dr. Wagner said.

Jason's skin was cold. His grip was strong. I clung to this branch, thinking about how even though I made it through the beginning of this appointment alone, I still needed him.

MAKING IT

The day my first pregnancy ended with Sophia's birth (and death), I was allowed to leave the hospital just thirteen hours later. The nurse, Jeanette, who had given me the discharge papers, had instructed me to take it easy for a few days, explained that I would continue to bleed until my uterus expelled all of its contents, that I could go ahead and resume drinking alcohol, that I should take Tylenol for any lingering soreness. She was the one who delivered our box of the only belongings that Sophia had: a cast of her (slightly larger than Barbie) hands, the dress the nurses put her in to take her birth photos, the disc of those photos, the blanket that protected her skin from ours, the tassel to her knit hat (one that would have fit a Beanie Baby), a poem about angels, her inky hand prints and foot prints.

Jeanette said, "take your time and you can leave when you are ready." She left us alone with the folder and the box.

Jason hugged me. He grabbed my hand with his left, holding Sophia's box with his right.

Sophia's body had already left the hospital, transported to the Milwaukee County coroner's office for the autopsy en route to the funeral home. Jason and I exited with all we had.

...

Studies have shown that couples who suffer miscarriage are twenty-two percent more likely to separate than those who have healthy, living babies. For those who have a stillbirth—the loss of a child who dies in the womb—separation of husband and wife is forty percent greater. The same forty percent applied to live births that devolve into death. Those are the babies who suffer the misfortune of having their genes mutated in such a way that the disfigurement of their hearts, or lungs, or brains, or intestines, or skin, or mouths, or hands, or knees, or ankles, or feet deem them nonviable with life. Just as my first and fourth pregnancies had been presumed to be.

...

After coming home from Sophia's birth, I took two weeks off work before I decided I needed to normalize my life. During those fourteen days, I drifted. The kitchen, the living room, the bedroom, our small backyard while pulling weeds from around our patio. I didn't want to see our neighbor, so I rarely ventured out. She knew we were expecting a baby. She was that middle-aged single neighbor that walked her dog daily while stopping to chat with every neighbor on the street. The Halloween before Sophia's birth, I popped outside onto our front porch to hand out candy to some children. Sitting on her own front step, she waved and said, "How are you and the baby?" I didn't know how I would answer that question anymore.

One day, Jason and I went to Target and bought a jigsaw puzzle. We spread out the pieces on our coffee table. Hours passed as we put together the pastel flowers.

Some days I spent reading *A Time to Decide, A Time to Heal-For Parents Making Difficult Decisions About Babies They Love*, a book compiled by two social workers and a medical doctor. It was the consolation prize the hospital sent home with us.

...

Marital separations often happen soon after the loss, with most occurring during the first one-and-a-half to three years. But passing year three does not guarantee relationships are safe. Up to ten years later, couples still fall victim to the damage that loss can befall on a relationship, the heartache that wedges between two people who were experimenting with grief. Jason and I weren't born knowing how to handle the loss of a child. How to handle naming a baby who wouldn't live more than an hour-and-a-half. It wasn't innate for me to watch Sophia lie in Jason's palms while loving her and awaiting her death. I hadn't learned how to respond when the doctor checked her heartbeat for the final time. Yet, Jason and I survived.

I couldn't look at the pictures we brought home from the hospital the day Sophia died, even when my family wanted to see them. I closed myself in the bedroom, laid on the bed, and hid my face in the comforter.

The first night home I was exhausted. Saved by my body's inability to stay awake any longer, I slept. Fitfully. When I woke in the morning, there was a moment, a single fraction of a second, in which I didn't remember that I had just given birth and lost a child the day before.

Once, years later when working at the neuropsychology clinic, I said to my coworker Karen: *I wonder if that is what it is like to have dementia. Do they feel a blissful lack of confusion, a moment in which they do not, or cannot, remember that they can't remember?*

Karen nodded. She knew what I meant.

But, unlike dementia, infant loss doesn't induce a lingering forgetfulness. The pain of the birth, the fear of seeing Sophia's tiny red body, the way her skin tore as she rolled on my chest, the slowing of her chest rising and falling, the doctor calling her time of death—remembering it all again was torture.

This remembering happened the next morning. And the next. And the next...

Within the sleep was insomnia. I fell asleep for an hour or two, but then would awake. I found my way to the couch. I turned on late-night TV. Some nights it wasn't too bad—Carson Daly's late-night show shifted my mind from how life sucked (how I wasn't sleeping and would be exhausted, how I just knew I'd never had children, how I kept realizing that I was now a mother to a deceased child) to current music trends. Peppy and sometimes obnoxious, the songs were not my life. I needed anything but my life.

Infomercials dominated the rest of the night. The one am, the two am, the three am. I learned about My Pillow™ and how it could contour your head and neck in the perfect way. It could help you sleep so soundly that you would feel rested *better than ever before!* It stayed cool while keeping you comfortable.

Would it also take away the pain? Would it allow *me* to sleep again?

I respected Jason's need for grieving in his way, although I was never sure what way that was. Sometimes he cried. Sometimes he just held me. Sometimes he didn't say much at all. I could always see his eyes moving back and forth, appearing like he was scanning the room for all the answers. I knew that face. It came out when he was thinking about a new proof for his math papers, or when he was thinking about a funny clip he found on Reddit, or when he was trying hard to not make a joke when I said words such as "balls" or "holes."

In the days following Sophia's death, and the other losses, I saw this face a lot. His eyes surveyed the floor (a lot). He appeared to be thinking (a lot). I never knew what was going on, but the pain on his face never wavered.

He noticeably became more emotional to others' plights. When a Facebook friend of his had a child born early and had to stay in the NICU, his eyes filled with tears. His voice choked. He needed a moment to calm the muscles in his jaw, the ones that pucker when crying is imminent. It made his chin quiver.

I never knew what he was thinking when his cheeks tensed or when his blue eyes watered. Yet I could *sense* the emotion. I could *feel* his sadness. It didn't matter to me which moment he was remembering, or wishing wasn't real. I was just glad I wasn't alone.

We both bought diaries. His: a plain black leather cover. Mine: tan with a blue and green bird and an art deco flower. I wrote letters to Sophia. I told her how beautiful she was (but not that I was scared to see her reddened skin, her bent limbs, her fragile body, her hairless scalp). I wrote of the moments I touched her (but not that I thought I ripped the red skin on her arm) and the words I whispered (*I love you, I'm so sorry, you are the best baby...*).

At night we sat up, side-by-side in bed, our journals on our laps.

Did you write in your journal? Oh, you did, that's good! No, no... you don't have to share. That's for you.

As much I wanted to know what he said to Sophia, (Was it: *I love you; Hello, I'm your daddy; I tried to save you; I did everything I could to help your mommy; You can rest now; If there was a God—and [he would add] I figured out over time there likely wasn't—but if there was, he would never let this happen to a baby; to MY baby*). I never looked in Jason's book.

SUPPORT GROUP

Before I was discharged from the maternity ward, a social worker suggested we attend a support group for bereaved parents. I didn't want to be there, sitting with strangers, in the very hospital where my first child, Sophia, had died. I didn't want to be in the same place where my baby was sitting in the cold box of the morgue, wrapped in plastic (I imagined) to keep her body from decomposing too much before the autopsy.

Just as I didn't want to wake up every morning, day after day, week after week, month after month, year after year, decade after decade, knowing that I was now a mother of a deceased child.

The fluorescent lights illuminated a ring of chairs. It was the middle of winter, and the window exposed a barren, snow-covered garden. People lined the outer edge of the room. Some sat with crumpled tissues, others looked at the floor, the window, the cup of coffee in their hands. No one was talking. Not yet.

It hadn't started *yet*.

...

The stench of grief was stubborn. It wouldn't disperse away from the people, away from the circle we created along the walls, away from the clock ticking on the wall, away from the coffee urn, away from this room, this hospital, this life.

I didn't want to venture inside further and contract the gloominess that permeated the room. If I didn't go inside, I couldn't be one of them.

When the discharge nurse had handed us the informational sheet about the Tuesday night support group (*meeting 6-8pm! Coffee served!*) I shoved it deep behind the other papers in the discharge folder and buried it just like the bodies of our young babies would be. Just like how I wanted my tears, my shallow sobbing breaths, my insomnia, and my thoughts of how impossible life would continue on to be.

If I couldn't see the flyer the nurse gave us, if I didn't drive to the Tuesday night support group, if I didn't walk into the lobby and follow the instructions from the information desk woman to walk down the hallway to the left, if I didn't pour a cup of coffee, open a little plastic creamer, or sit down, then I wasn't one of them.

...

Does it matter where we sit? Are there some veterans here who have 'their chair' and would be upset if I came in and disrupted their pattern? Disrupted their desperate clinging to whatever stability they could find, even if it was a chair, week in and week out?

Jason and I had taken the seats closest to the door. I wanted a quick escape in case the meeting became unbearable. I wanted a quick escape in case they started to make me feel like I was one of them. In case I remembered too much of what happened. In case I started to believe it.

...

For the first time in five days, I didn't have to disclose that my daughter had died. That I wasn't the mother I thought I would be, that I couldn't save my own child. I didn't have to explain to anyone sitting in the circle that I *was* pregnant and was *no longer* pregnant, or why I had no child to show for it.

These were basic requirements for admittance.

...

My fingers anxiously played with the fringes of my scarf. A gnawing feeling in my gut screamed. *Cut your losses, dash back home through the snowy evening, and cry your tears in private!*

Like people do. Behind closed doors.

...

At this point, I had worked in mental health for eight years. I held a bachelor's degree in psychology and a master's in clinical psychology. I worked with children who suffered from ADHD, autism, learning disorders, and mood dysregulation. I helped patients in treatment facilities. I tested their abilities with our proven psychological assessments.

I believed in it all—the cognitive behavioral therapies and the medications and the true nature of mental health issues. All as real as heart disease or diabetes or cancer or the chicken pox that had riddled my young five-year-old skin all those years ago, a single scar left near my belly button.

Yet…how could I possibly benefit from hearing what others have gone through?

How could I *not*?

...

Anxiety created regular nightmares. Dreams twisted into wild imagery.

My dreams were so life-like that I had trouble distinguishing them from my waking hours. As a child, I dreamt of my grandparents at the checkout line of Target. As they paid the cashier, my grandmother's arms popped off on springs and my grandfather's eyeballs fell out in a bloody mess. The fear startled me awake. It took several minutes of adjusting my eyes to the dimness of the early morning light before I regained my reality. No one had really died. No blood ran from the bodies of two people I held dear.

Now, as an adult, I sat here unsure of which world I was in. I felt awake. Jason sat next to me. His fingers wrapped around mine. The hardness of the chair pushed into the back of my thighs; the edge of the seat dug through my jeans. The burnt coffee behind me made me want to vomit. The perishing fetus I had carried, the birth that came too early, the death. It all seemed so real. But then again, so did the grotesque way my grandparents had "died."

I noted each look of pain on the faces that lined the circle. Each sullen face: cheeks sunken, eyes darkened, lips downturned. Each person whose head hung low to make fleeting eye contact at best. *Why were they here? To understand what had happened? Or to understand* ***why****?*

I wanted to know if this was another terrible dream, if we existed at all.

...

We sat in a room with six other couples.

I fingered a tissue that was waiting in my pocket, just in case.

I looked at the floor.

Here we go, I thought.

Facilitator

"Let's go ahead and begin," a woman said. Her purple scrubs and tired eyes described her long day of nursing. My mother-in-law was a nurse, and I recognized that "just worked a twelve-hour shift" face. Yet here was this woman, offering up two more hours of her day to sit with this sad circle, badge dangling from her breast pocket. I bowed my head and listened.

"I see some new faces tonight," she said, "so let's all take a turn and introduce ourselves. Feel free to say whatever you feel comfortable saying about yourself."

She was talking about me. About Jason and me and our lost Sophia.

I looked around. I dared to look at each face, even when they didn't reciprocate.

Who are these people who lost their babies?

Where did they come from, why do we never hear about them?

And, most frighteningly, how did I become one of them?

"Let's begin with you please, if you don't mind," the nurse said. She pointed to a couple who sat directly across from her, two away from us.

Twin Loss

The couple spoke of their twin boys.

"We lost both of them, for no known medical reason," the woman said. "We had a nursery for them, we were so excited. And then it was over, and they were gone forever." I saw the tear drops spreading into dark circles on the thighs of her jeans. "Just as I lost my babies, I feel like I lost my emotional control."

Neither one was her fault, I knew. But just as I considered what I could have done differently to save my baby, did she do this, too?

"We planted two trees in our garden to remember them," the woman said.

What if those trees die, too?

Necklace of Ashes

"It was the day the ladies in my office threw me a baby shower. They had everything decorated and brought in food. It was so nice," she smiled briefly.

"Yet, I couldn't enjoy it because I began feeling sick. I did my best to open all the gifts and appear to be having a good time, but by the end of the party, I had to go home to rest. Since I was eight months along," she swallowed hard, "no one thought it was strange that I needed this down time. By the next day, however, I was in the hospital, going into pre-term labor. She didn't survive the virus I contracted." She paused.

"Our baby died that day."

She lost her seemingly healthy baby at eight months.

Eight months.

Eight months of thinking everything was okay.

Eight months of preparing for a healthy baby girl.

Eight months of watching sonograms and hearing heartbeats.

Eight months of blissful ignorance of how bad it could be.

Her husband squeezed her left hand. Her right hand busied itself twisting a small charm on her necklace.

She paused and took a breath before speaking.

"I keep thinking, what if I didn't get sick? Did I not wash my hands enough? Did I not rest enough?" Her words accelerated as if her thoughts were on a train speeding out of control down the tracks. "*What did I do wrong?!*" Spitting out these final words, her train fell over the edge of the cliff. No tracks left to hold her up.

I couldn't stop watching the necklace, how she smoothed it between her thumb and index finger.

Her husband, who had been silent until this point, quietly spoke: "We were blindsided by this. Everything was going along so well. My wife was healthy. The baby was healthy. And then something went horribly wrong. But I know it's not her fault. It's nobody's fault. There was nothing we could have done differently to prevent this. The doctor said so."

The woman had regained her composure, barely. She pulled at the necklace charm as far as the chain would let it extend. It was tiny, gold (I think). Sitting across the circle from her, I couldn't see what it was—a heart, a little bear, something else?

"This necklace contains the last trace of our baby. We had a little bit of her ashes put in this charm. I cannot take it off. I wear it all the time. When I'm sleeping. When I'm in the shower. Always. I don't know what I would do if I ever took it off."

Thank goodness I'm not like that, I'm not looking for something to cling to. If I don't have a necklace like that, then I can't be like her.

She pulled out an e-reader from her bag.

"The only other thing we have of her is a picture we took shortly after she was born." Her finger swiped the screen, scrolling for a full minute. Looking at the screen, she passed it to the right. I had done a good job of maintaining my poker face until that point. Through her story. Through her husband's quiet confessions. Through the horror of what happens to everyday people. People—adults—who are someone's children, someone's friends, and now someone's parent.

Oh, shit, I thought as the tablet made it to the woman next to me.

When the tablet came to me, my face crumbled. At first, it seemed like an image of a content, sleeping, perfect baby girl. She wore a flowered dress and matching headband. I knew this picture was not what it seemed. She was not sleeping.

Seven Miscarriages

A man, attending alone, explained that he and his wife have had seven miscarriages.

I had only had one at this point, so I could certainly not be as bad off as him. That is what I wanted to be: not as bad as him. Not as bad as all the people I was sitting with.

"We had truly been lost for what to do," he said, "I've been coming for the past five years. My wife isn't here because she just couldn't bear to come anymore. I can't blame her. I just don't know how to stop."

Then he said, "we decided to adopt instead. We now have a little boy."

What the hell? Does he have the right to be here, to speak after we just looked at a necklace that was the final resting place for another?

We all smiled as best as we could. We nodded as he passed around a picture of the child.

I hated him for sharing this picture. For sharing this kind of news. I was in no mood to hear of a happy adoption, nor of how he and his wife finally had the child they so longed for.

My child died five days ago.

Through my psychological training to watch people's faces, their body positioning, their arms and legs crossed or not, I was usually a good read of people.

This room was particularly difficult to decipher.

I looked adoringly (or at least I tried) at the picture and passed it on to Jason. He quickly gave it to the man next to him.

Watching his face sink, his cheeks hollowing even more into his narrow jawline, I thought about how our loss has changed *Jason*. I had known him for nearly ten years, and I had never seen him cry so much. I had never seen him tear up over a picture of someone *else's* kid. I had never seen him so choked up he was unable to get the words he wanted to say out into the open. Now, I had seen this repeatedly. He was a changed man. *Have seven miscarriages changed this other man even more?*

Molar Pregnancy

We continued around the room. A woman, attending alone, talked of her two failed pregnancies. A molar pregnancy and a miscarriage. She described how a molar pregnancy was a group of cells that grew but did not form an actual life being.

"There was a possibility of the cell cluster becoming cancerous," she added.

It was a *cancer*?

The *baby* was a *cancer*.

A tumor that replaced what should have been a new life was instead a threat to this woman's health. How can a baby—what should be the miracle of life—be, in fact, a nightmare?

Thank goodness Sophia wasn't a cancerous cell bunch.

Or was she (in her own way)?

I admired the courage this woman had.

It felt selfish to be thankful at a time like this.

She was an engineer. And while she attended alone, she confessed she was in a stable marriage. She did not talk about her husband beyond the initial reference.

Was her husband ashamed?

Was their marriage threatened at the loss, volatile fights erupting where they once didn't belong?

Or was he scared? Scared of being one of them?

Like me?

The engineer seemed so normal. I imagined her husband would be, too. Grief seemed to take on many faces. Her husband was not ready to be here. Perhaps he felt that if he didn't attend, his baby won't have been a bunch of fast-growing cells that could have killed his wife.

She had suffered. Maybe she suffered more than we had. Sure, we were both college-educated, married, employed, stable. We looked to be about the same age. But my story was not *hers*. I couldn't possibly look as she did, defeated by life.

Yet, the more I heard, the more I knew I had suffered, too.

Near Death of the Mother

The next couple was quiet, like Jason and me. They never removed their coats. I wondered if they were also planning a quick escape. They seemed to be in their early twenties. Quietly, barely above a whisper, they talked about how recently it had happened and how fresh the emotions were.

The man talked about how he was so scared at the hospital, not only because he was losing his baby, but also because watching his wife hemorrhage meant he had to worry about losing her, too. He began to cry, which made Jason cry. Then I cried. Others, too.

Jason leaned over and softly confessed to only me, "I know exactly how that man feels. I knew we were going to lose our baby, but I don't know what I'd do if I also lost you."

The only way our situation would be worse is if we didn't have each other. But I had never realized that Jason had lived this fear. My heart sank impossibly lower. It sagged to the floor kicking around between my wet boots on the dingy hospital carpet. A couple of fresh tears joined in.

Angry Couple

The woman sitting next to Jason was angry. I couldn't follow her words through the yelling, the reddened face, the tears that accompanied her harsh tone. I couldn't follow what had happened to her pregnancy, how far along she was, how long ago it had happened, how many baby items they had bought before the loss. All I knew was the loss had made her angry.

Her husband seemed angry, too, but quieter about it. Perhaps he was letting his wife vent and saved his for at home. Perhaps he didn't know how to be angry like her. Perhaps he didn't know quite what to feel.

But *she* was angry.

At least I'm not like her.

Twenty-Week Loss

It was our turn. Jason and I held hands as we looked to each other and tried to figure out who would talk first.

I cleared my throat and started to say, "My name is Laura. And this is Jason. We just recently..." my throat choked up cutting off any passage for air. I stared at the floor, tried to breathe deeply and collect myself. I failed. I could feel all eyes on me as *my* sorrow became overwhelmed by other people's sorrow. Jason picked up where I left off. Since our early days together, he's always had my back. If I was short on money, he picked up the tab. If I let my nerves get the best of me while going to a new restaurant or meeting a new person, he put himself ahead of me to lead the way. And now, when words were impossible to extract from my throat, my tongue sodden with saliva, he stepped up.

"We lost our baby last Friday," he said. "We don't know what happened. We were told it was probably a genetic disorder," he said. I stared at the floor. I was grateful. I couldn't bear the embarrassment of crying in front of all these strangers for much longer.

Can we just move on and let someone else speak?

Jason told of how difficult it was to tell others our story. How we felt we let our families, our friends, and everyone down. Then, for the remainder of the two hours, we sat and listened.

And we cried.

I cried for myself. I cried for Jason. I cried for having a reason to be here in the first place. I cried for not feeling angry like the couple on the other side of Jason did. I cried for feeling too numb. I cried for being too sad. I cried for not being sad enough. I cried for crying too much.

I cried because I fit in with those who had gone before. It was the only support group we attended. I couldn't sit in the grief of others for two hours every Tuesday night.

As soon as Jason and I left the room, I never had to see them again. The engineer, the twin–loss couple, the woman with the necklace, the man with his adopted son.

I could be nothing like them.

I could go home and separate myself again.
Except that I couldn't unhear their stories.

GENERALIZED ANXIETY DISORDER (GAD)

When I was twenty-five, I sat in my favorite graduate course on child psychopathology. It was where I first read about Generalized Anxiety Disorder. The DSM-IV TR, *the* manual for the disorders of the human mind, laid open to page four-hundred seventy-two, diagnosis number 300.02 Generalized Anxiety Disorder (GAD) (Includes Overanxious Disorder of Childhood).

Other students were arriving and taking their seats, but as I sat in the second row from the front of the room, up against a wall, where not many could see what I was doing. Dr. Papadakous's youthful style was easy-going and informative. She sorted through her lecture notes on the day's topic of anxiety disorders. I wanted to be calm, assured, and steady, too.

I looked over the criteria again. When I had read the GAD section previously, I had highlighted only the first line, the one that summarized the first requirement as 'excessive worry' or 'apprehensive expectation' that is more common than not, extending more months than not.

Could this be me? I had thought.

Dr. Papadakous began, "Okay, class. Let's begin our discussion of anxiety disorders that can present in childhood. What do we know about panic attacks and how they relate to agoraphobia?"

She started on page four-hundred thirty of the anxiety disorders section, but I couldn't wait to get back to GAD.

The 'familial pattern' section for GAD, one that is always included for disorders and describes just how much a genetic component may contribute to the presentation, starts with "Anxiety as a trait has a familial association."

Could this be my mom?

Could I have gotten this from her?

And if so, what did that matter?

Could this just be who we are, her and me, two genetically connected people who share body types, standing postures, wavy hair, and an overactive brain?

...

I knew that self-diagnosis was a dangerous thing.

Yet, I couldn't help but wonder why I matched every criterion. I disliked having to navigate how to meet new people; making phone calls to people I could not see when talking (because watching their lips move when talking is crucial...what if I can't hear them? What if they don't enunciate? What if they have crooked teeth? What if they smile and I don't know they are smiling and I think they are serious and I feel bad?); walking into new situations like new schools, new jobs, moving into a new home with new neighbors; the prospect of failing and the fear that I *had* failed. I worried about what people thought of my hair, my voice, what I said, how I looked, my jokes, my personality. I would practice hypothetical conversations with people just so I knew exactly how it might go (or how I imagined they would go, but likely wouldn't). I replayed conversations that already happened, chiding myself for not saying something different, something better, something wittier, or clever, or smart. Worrying about every detail, even the unimportant ones, was overwhelming. Even the smallest of chores or to-do lists made me want to shut my brain down and take a nap.

But I never thought buried within how I was, what I thought, or how I behaved there might be something wrong.

Or that others lived differently.

Or that I was part of a small group of people who reportedly felt "anxious and nervous all their lives."

Or that there is a high likelihood of a genetic association with others in my family who also live with high levels of anxiety.

Or that my own mother may have grown up with similar fears, or that I would grow up to exhibit her current behaviors.

Or that I was likely also playing out learned behaviors alongside the genes that crippled my sympathetic nervous system—the fight-or-flight response.

I didn't consider that I was part of the five percent of people reported to have GAD over the course of a lifetime.

I never considered that I *could* live differently.

...

Insight, as I discovered through my DSM and through Dr. Papadakous, gave me hope that what I noticed in my mom, in myself, in the traits that we both had, in the habits that had been passed down and behaviorally learned, was not predestined. When *I* have a child, I could let them play with my stuffed bear Biggie without worrying when his tongue rips out or his holes get bigger. When that child leaves Legos, pennies spilled from a piggy bank, and Little People figures all over their bedroom floor, I could sit on the carpet and help them clear the space again without feeling overwhelmed by the mess—without making *them* feel overwhelmed. When that child grows up and goes to the movies with friends on a Friday evening after eating dinner at the local Applebee's, I won't care enough about laundry to leave them reminder notes to put their laundry out the night before I plan to wash it. I won't sort my laundry into so many piles. Or only two piles: light and dark (because it still made sense to not bleed colors). When my child starts kindergarten, middle school, high school, or has a new teacher, new friends, new coursework, or learns to drive, goes on a first date, gets asked to prom, moves away to college, signs up to study abroad, graduates, goes on job interviews, gets married, has their own child, I could tell them *it will all work out.*

Maybe by then, ten years in the future, I will believe that, too.

CRITERIA I NEED TO MEET TO SELF-DIAGNOSE (PART 1 OF 4)[4]

Criterion 1: The essential feature of Generalized Anxiety Disorder is excessive anxiety and worry (apprehensive expectation), occurring more days than not for a period of at least six months about a number of events.

I was about five years old and my closet was a mess. When my mom found it, she asked me to clean it up. I cried. I sat on the floor, frozen. Where do I start? The idea of finding a place for all of the toys, the shirts, and the stuffed animals, having to fold the socks into the little ball bundles my mom liked, putting the dirty socks and underwear into the shared hamper that was in my sister's room, that was all too much.

It wasn't a large closet as we lived in a small ranch-style house that was cookie-cutter to those others built around us in the 1980s.

---

[4] Bruises accumulated on my legs, and I decided I had leukemia. (source: a YA fiction book, title not remembered-- *not important?*); I started driving and felt that my eyesight was worse during night driving, and I determined I had a degenerative eye disease that appeared at night before progressing to complete blindness (source: YA book titled "Tiger Eyes"); I started having headaches that made my eyeballs feel inflated making them too big for their sockets, and I determined I had migraines, or cluster headaches, or just tension headaches? (source: WebMD, Wikipedia, Google, personal blogs). Once I considered that I had hypochondriasis (assigning myself diagnoses that weren't true) but then I wondered: *could a hypochondriac self-diagnose hypochondriasis?*

It had shelves up high, a wooden pole that I couldn't yet reach, and a floor that stretched deep back. The floor was the space I used. I shoved my stuffed animals in there when my mom asked me to clean my room. Biggie was my favorite teddy bear, his fur still soft and his original pink tongue stuck out of his slightly opened mouth. I was mortified that now the closet floor held so much more than just him.

"Let's do this together," my mom had said when she found me. "I'll help you this time."

She got down next to me. She began pulling out all the things, one at a time, asking me where it should go. We put the stuffed animals back in the homes that I had been asked to designate for them: the small ones on the bookshelf, the larger ones in a corner piled neatly with their faces showing, and Biggie on my bed. My dirty clothes were piled for their trip to the hamper in Sarah's room. The clean single socks were lined up with their match, then rolled and tucked. The clean shirts were refolded: first placed front-side down, one sleeve at a time folded onto the back of the shirt, then doubled-over onto itself again before folding the entire shirt in half. I would have rolled them up, haphazardly tucking in the sleeves, but when folding with my mom (or for my mom, or next to my mom) that was not okay.

The piles were then put away in the dresser drawers.

"Pull with both handles," my mom said as I grabbed only one metal ring. I put the stack of shirts down that I had balanced carefully on my forearm and pulled with two hands. I didn't understand why. It was the same with any drawer in my dressers, the lid to the piano keys, or the sliding doors that covered the thirteen-inch TV that always had to be tucked back away in its living room armoire when we were done watching our allotted thirty minutes of cartoons, or reality shows of the time like "Rescue 911" and "Unsolved Mysteries."

Both shows caused me to fear that something bad would happen to me, to my family, to my home. According to Robert Stack, the host of "Unsolved Mysteries," there were murderers still out there lurking in people's windows and aliens that continue coming down and taking people on mysterious half-remembered missions. The worst episode showed one man whose shoulder just caught on fire as he stood in his kitchen. This is how I learned the term spontaneous combustion.

I didn't know how to not think that our home would be broken into or that I'd be shot at by a killer on the loose. This was a fear that lingered with me into adulthood—if Robert Stack didn't know where these bad people were, why wouldn't they be lurking in the bushes at my apartment complex as I walked my dog one last time before going to bed?

This particular afternoon, however, I didn't worry about my leg catching on fire.

With my mom's help, the closet floor came back.

"Good work, Laura," my mom said. "Now try to keep it this way and you won't have to clean it like that again."

I wanted to keep it pristine forever. But when my childhood messiness threatened orderliness, I didn't know how to make them coexist.

For now, there was harmony. Harmony between my floor and my toys, the dirty laundry and the hamper, my mom's sense of peace and my nervousness.

I could smile again. What should I play with next? Where was my sister? How do I pass the next chunk of the day?

I found Sarah in her room.

"Wanna play, Sarah?"

"Okay. What do you want to play with?"

We pulled out the old Barbies that had belonged to my mom and her sister.

...

"You can play with these as long as you take care of them, which means you put them away when you are done with them. Okay?" my mom said the day she brought her Barbies out from their box in the basement.

We carefully took them out of their cases, the ones from the sixties that opened like standing suitcases and held all of Barbie's clothes and accessories. We brushed Barbie's hair gently because loose strands should not come out; pulled on and off her clothing slowly so as not to rip any seams; accounted for every shoe, every tiny earring that fit through the tiny holes in her lobes, and every clip-on necklace. When we were done playing, we were mindful to place them and their accessories back in their cases: the tiny blouses, the skirts, the small black cat-eye glasses.

There were few items saved from my parents' childhoods. I sensed that as much as my mom wanted to preserve the integrity of her old toys and of the thirty-one-year-old memories she had with her own sister, she also wanted to share a piece of herself with Sarah and me. The Barbie boxes were musty when opened, revealing age, dust, and the careful preservation my mother had for her belongings, even as a child.

These dolls were how she bonded with her sister. Now they were how I bonded with mine. Even while she worried about the well-being of the dolls, she trusted us with a piece of her life.

We just had to be careful.

We always had to be careful.

Criterion 2: The individual finds it difficult to control the worry.

I avoid: social activities, small talk (because I'll second-guess my conversations and actions for hours afterward), and eating in front of others (in case a piece of spinach gets stuck between my teeth, or chicken wing sauce makes a rim around my lips, or a speck of basil sticks to my mouth). I worry I will fail at anything I try, like going to college; any change in my comfortable routine induces my intestines to cramp and my stomach to threaten a vomiting episode. Anything that others may find exciting—going on a vacation, starting a new class, meeting friends for happy hour—make me fearful. Yet, I always power through because I can't not.

Is that normal?

I've tried: deep breathing, forcing my thoughts to happier things, smiling on the outside when I'm not smiling on the inside, tensing my facial muscles so I don't frown, don't grimace, don't scream, don't cry.

Nothing seems to work.

Criterion 3: The anxiety, worry, or physical symptoms cause clinically significant distress or impairment in social, occupational, or other important areas of functioning.

The first day of school was terrifying. I was entering fourth grade where everything would be different. My teacher was going to be the first male teacher I ever had: Mr. Ritonia. Even though kids in Sarah's grade a year ahead of me thought he was the "cool teacher," I wasn't sure. I didn't know how to get to know him after a whole year with Mrs. Oudenhoven, a towering older woman who wore ankle-length black sweaters that matched her permed salt-and-pepper hair. Sarah had had Mrs. O before me. Mrs. O was familiar. I didn't have much to learn about her after hearing the stories of her spelling tests from my sister, and how she handed out stickers for perfect scores. She was the teacher whom I was excited to show my first rejection letter from a publishing house after I tried to pitch my handmade book on dinosaurs.

"Oh, how exciting that you got a letter in the mail!" Mrs. O had said.

But now, the eve before fourth grade, I couldn't sleep. The fourth graders were on a different side of the building—in the green learning center. I would no longer be in the blue one. They were paired with the red learning center—the one that housed the bigger fifth graders.

Would they make fun of me? I wondered.

They are so old!

They are the crossing guards outside!

They run this school.

I wanted to know which kids would be in my classroom. I had had a best friend, Jenny, in the first and second grade, but by the time we went to third grade, she had become best friends with Alison instead. They no longer talked to me. I didn't know how to make a new best friend. There was the boy, Tommy, who wore the same Bart Simpson shirt and gray sweatpants every day. He smelled of stale body odor and was seemingly into a TV show I wasn't allowed to watch. There was another boy, Pete, who broke his collarbone and had a large cast that spanned up his arm and across his shoulders. He would later be seated in my grouping of four desks, right across from me in Mr. Ritonia's class, and I would be the one to help him pick up his pencil when it dropped and get his schoolwork out of his desk.

The uncertainty of Mr. Ritonia's room, the green learning center, the kids I knew from third grade but who weren't in Mrs. O's room, and having to see Jenny and Alison be friends all kept me from sleeping. I came out of my room after my dad had put me to bed. He had kissed my forehead, as always. The sheet came up to my shoulders. I always covered my arms to hide them from the scary murderers running loose that "Unsolved Mysteries" told me about. It was summer with no air conditioning, too warm for my comforter, which my dad folded neatly half-way down the bed. *I'll make it so you can reach the edge in case you want it*, he told me. By the time I came out of my room my parents were sitting on the couch watching a late-night program. The green plastic bowl sat on the coffee table, a sign that they had made popcorn.

"What's wrong, Laura?" my mom asked.

I walked up to her and sat on her lap. I cried.

"Is it school tomorrow?"

I nodded. How did she know? I tried to be fine at dinner; we ate sitting at our unofficially assigned chairs at the table, I had two servings of spaghetti—one with sauce and second with just parmesan cheese—we slid our plates through the small sliding door my dad had built between the wall that divided the dining room and the kitchen. I didn't talk about school. I let the thoughts of friends, teachers, and new classrooms, desks, and learning center colors live only in my mind.

"Blueberry, Blueberry, what am I going to do-berry?" she said after a long silence. She folded me into her crocheted Afghan, wrapping me in soft orange and green and brown.

Being called 'Blueberry' always calmed me when I was upset and made me laugh harder when I was being silly.

I sat with my mom for several more minutes. I knew things would be new and scary and different tomorrow, but I would come home to this.

THE TROLL IN THE LAUNDRY ROOM

I was in the basement laundry room watching my mom take clothes from the laundry basket and sort them into piles: whites, lights, darks, and jeans. The old machines were the color of flower pollen—a yellow only suitable for the 1980s. They were hidden in a room that took three turns from the bottom of the stairs and passed the large drawing table my mom used for her airbrushing and painting. It felt like a maze, like the bright yellow machines were hidden away in the farthest corner of the house, yet they held so much importance. The piles surrounded me: whites for a bleach load, light colors together for warm water, dark colors for the cold wash. Jeans were never put in the dryer and always ironed. I watched this ritual with fascination, always wondering how she never felt like it was too much work to do. I thought, *so much sorting! How does she remember all this? Is it ever done?*

At one point, my mother left the room. "I'll be right back, Laura, okay? You stay right here." I watched her walk off into the art room and turn left back into the darker part of the basement. I didn't dare leave the bright lights of the fluorescent bulbs, the ones that kept away all the scary things that I believed lived on the other side of the basement—the side with the packed boxes of old dishes, skis and poles too big for boxes, and deer hides from my father's hunting days. I instead stayed near the machines. It was the last place I knew I felt safe before she left me there alone. I opened the brown metal cabinet, one that towered over me. It was the food pantry as our small kitchen couldn't fit anything beyond our plates and bowls and utensils. Even the television (a five-inch GE portable TV/Radio) had to hang from underneath the cabinets to save what little yellow counter space there was. In the brown metal cabinet, the garbanzo beans were stacked, the Spam sat in a row, and the boxes of mac and cheese were lined up like army men ready to battle in the kitchen. Each label faced outward. "So I can easily see what everything is," my mom often explained.

When she returned, she asked me to look in her back pocket. "I think something might be in there. Can you check?" Sticking out of the denim of her high-waisted jeans was a tuft of gray and white hair. It was attached to a head, plastic the color of flesh. I pulled at the hair. "Careful!" my mom said. "He's old and I don't want the hair to come off." The troll slid out easily. He was naked. His belly button and googly eyes made me giggle.

"He's for you now," my mom told me. "I thought you might like him."

He was ugly. His smile made me feel safe. I hugged my mom's stone-washed denimed legs.

"Thanks, Mommy," I said.

Over the years, I became intrigued with troll dolls. I collected many: large ones with stuffed bodies and removable clothing, tiny ones that sat on top of pencils, ones with rainbow hair and ones with pink hair, and an extra fat one with purple hair. All except the gray-haired one have since been donated to Goodwill.

THE ODDS

One-in-four pregnancies end in miscarriage. That means that most people I knew had either experienced a loss or knew someone who did. Until I lost Sophia, I did not know how rampant it was. It was like cancer. I knew several people who had fought cancer, died from cancer, or were people who knew other people who had cancer.

We talk about cancer.

My mom's friend Terry died of pancreatic cancer. Patrick Swayze, too. My Uncle Keith died of kidney cancer. I have now had two co-workers who had breast cancer (and survived!), and another whose spouse was diagnosed with lung cancer. It had been rumored that Val Kilmer had throat cancer. Michael Douglas contracted mouth (or was it tongue?) cancer from Catherine Zeta-Jones.

Miscarriage, like cancer, was everywhere. And once you experienced it, or knew someone who received the diagnosis, you were part of the club.

We don't talk about miscarriage.

When Sophia died, I worked as a psychometrist, administering psychological testing batteries to children and adult patients. I had seen children suffering from autism, their parents desperate for a way to connect with a child who wouldn't look them in the eye or say the words "I love you, Mommy." I tested patients who were in their fifties and were beginning to get lost when going to the store or couldn't remember what a spouse had told them five minutes prior. Early Onset Alzheimer's—the evil cousin of the more common

Alzheimer's Disease that affects the elderly—is genetic, and within two or three years, would debilitate an otherwise vibrant, healthy, prime-of-their-life adult. My days were filled with patients like this. But there was always hope of helping even some. Even just *one*. It was the reason I showed up day after day.

I never thought I'd be coming into the office being the bereaved one. *My coworkers will understand my situation,* I thought. I didn't expect just how much they understood. We had talked about our kids, and my bosses' son's boy scout camping trip, and the preschool teachers the other psychologists' children had, and even the adoption of one of the secretary's—now grown—children. But we had never talked about pregnancy loss before. Why would we?

One psychologist approached me and revealed he and his wife lost a child to Turner's syndrome. I had no idea what that was. When I got home, I Googled it. Just as I had searched for every one of Sophia's abnormalities and suspected conditions, I had to know.

Affects 1 in 2000 females, according to WebMD. *A female is missing an X chromosome. Children can live but may have a short stature.*

But his child hadn't lived. His daughter was in the same place as Sophia.

I had no idea that his perfect family, one that included a son and daughter, also included this other child. *Dr. Powell survived*, I had thought. *And he seems so normal.*

I was sitting in the office of the child psychologist who interviewed me for the job as her right-hand-person when she said, "I wanted to check in with you. Are you sure you are ready to come back to work? You know, before I had Lily, I had a miscarriage. Not that it is the same as your loss, but I just want you to know that I get it."

I began a blog four months after Sophia was born. People I went to high school with sent messages over social media. *I, too, had a loss between my second and third child,* they would say. Or sometimes it was a string of losses. Other times it was on their first try.

A friend of Jason's from college sent me a personal message detailing his and his wife's loss of their daughter. Another friend of Jason's, this one from high school, told me about his stillborn child. Both of these friends I had only known in name and through stories. Yet, they bore what I suspected was their darkest secret with *me*. A near stranger. It made me wonder just how intense our desire was to share what is otherwise unspeakable.

Through these stories, I made connections. A lot of connections. I felt the web of loss that quietly stretches across humanity. Its sinewy strings attached to each new person, new couple, new bereaved parent. Like the strength of the spiderwebs I've seen blowing in the gustiest of winds, the strings don't let go. Not even when a wind comes through threatening the adhesive bonds.

Spider webs are five times stronger than steel (if steel was made into the same thin fibers). Made up of nanofibers, each string—which is already one-thousand times *thinner* than a human hair—is made up of thousands of even tinier strands. These strands are woven around each other in complex ways. In fact, it is so complex that until recently, researchers could only hypothesize this was how spiders' webs worked. Now, using an atomic force microscope, and by looking exclusively at the web of a brown recluse spider (whose webs are flatter than others and therefore more easily seen under the atomic force microscope) they have confirmed their suspicions.

If researchers could put the connections between bereaved parents under the atomic force microscope, I wonder if the bonds would have the same strength. If they could capture the grief of watching a child die in your arms, or witness the heart go from beating one week to not beating the next, or give birth to a child already formed—eyes, nose, mouth, fingers, toes, and a set of lungs that no longer breathe. If they could then bolster a mother who held her child as he took his last breath and went limp in the palm of her hand. If they could make a father feel less helpless when his wife's doctor says, *I can't find the heartbeat.*

I built my strings. I talked about Sophia to my coworkers. I wrote on my blog about the details of her birth, her death, and her tiny facial features. I spoke her name every day. I wove together the nanothreads of people (coworkers, friends, close relatives, distant relatives, acquaintances, strangers) into a strand much stronger than myself. These connections kept me moving through the long hours at work, preparing dinners for our family of two, walking our happy-go-lucky dog, and waking up each morning only to relive the nightmare. This web kept me from curling up under my blanket and wishing each day was different.

The web of people did more than give strength. It showed a glimpse of a place where grief, loss, family, children, smiles, kindness, professional success, and positivity *all* existed.

…

Pregnancy revealed I had a uterine abnormality, either a septated uterus or a bicornuate one (no doctor really could tell me which). I had yet another thing to search on the Internet. It had a relatively rare occurrence, showing up in only about three percent of women. It can only be properly identified through MRI, which I hesitated to do. I didn't want the colored ink flowing into my uterus. I didn't want someone peering into my belly (again). I didn't want another invasion of my insides, one that would likely, I was sure, determine that I was guilty.

Guilty, not of intentionally making the only home my babies knew incompatible with growing a life, but guilty of *something*.[5]

...

Surgeons can remove the septation (a small flap of skin that divides the uterus nearly in two), but it may cause scar tissue that could increase the risk of future miscarriage. When this procedure was suggested to me, I already had endured a second miscarriage. I didn't know it at the time, but I would later add another loss to the count. *Would a risky procedure really put me on the winning side?*

...

Even with only three to seven percent of us affected, message boards filled with other women also faced with this dilemma: three to seven percent of women with a uterine septation (the most common type called a Müllerian anomaly[6]— *what I have?*), three to seven percent of us shared our guilt, our worry, our disappointment with our bodies. We only constitute three to seven percent of women, but when concentrated into one outlet, we seemed mighty.

Women got the surgery. Women warned against it. Still, some women were quick to tell their own success stories, wishing the rest of us *best of luck!* My life had already been turned upside down once Sophia's problems became apparent. I saw high-risk doctors, I braved

---

[5] Dr. Tamar Gur, M.D., PhD., a reproductive psychiatrist at The Ohio State University Wexner Medical Center, said *the guilt is common, but often misplaced*. Dr. Gur, along with others in her field, work to help women understand that miscarriage is usually unavoidable. The trouble is getting past the idea that held on strong after learning about my misshapen uterus: *my body failed this baby. It was my job, only I could do this, and I [my uterus] failed*.

[6] Other Müllerian anomalies: unicornuate uterus (under-developed duct, banana-shaped), a missing kidney or kidney issues (rare, but that's nitpicking...), uterus didelphys (a duplication of vagina, uterus, cervix).

long ultrasounds, I was advised to consider termination. The second pregnancy started out high-risk. I had many factors against me, against the baby. I spent my days wondering *how could this be?*

...

The subchorionic hematomas began during my second pregnancy. Another new diagnosis, another thing to fear. About one percent of pregnancies have this complication. Bleeding in the bathroom at work, on the couch at home, during the middle of the night, clots dislodging when they feel it is time to let go, to gush, to make me think I was losing more than just blood.

With all the odds coming true, and not having anything 'normal,' I began to wonder how it could be that these odds were stacked against me. If I had been gambling with an ante of an embryo and the desired outcome of miscarriage, I would be winning. In Las Vegas, if I had bet on a number in roulette, the odds would be against me. To choose a number straight up on the wheel, my odds of winning would be 2.9 percent. Better than having subchorionic hematomas, worse than having a septated uterus. I should have taken my misfortune to Vegas where it could have become something better.

...

Recurrent pregnancy loss, meaning a loss of three or more consecutive pregnancies, occurs in one to two percent of the female population, according to studies published on the National Institute of Health website. Before we lost our second pregnancy, I hadn't considered that subsequent pregnancies wouldn't work. When the ultrasound revealed all of Sophia's physical anomalies, with a condition 'likely not compatible with life,' we were also told it was 'likely a fluke.' *Chromosomes and genes can mutate, become deleted or corrupted*, the genetic counselor, Julie, had told us.

...

We had lived in San Diego after my third loss, for one year, when Jason was offered a visiting assistant professor job. It was a dream year for him, to work with a mathematician esteemed in his field. During this year we visited the beach. We dipped our toes into the water's edge. We never dared to venture too far from the sand that squeezed between our toes. I had read about rip currents. About people being swept away from shore. I imagined it felt like my first loss, when suddenly a rip current pulled one's feet out from underneath them and scraped their feet along the jagged coral. My feet were pulled out from beneath me. Julie, the genetic counselor, had the job of trying to convince me to swim with the current to survive. I had been doing what was normally advised: swim parallel to the beach to stay safe. I followed all the rules of pregnancy. I saw my doctor regularly. I only ate foods that would provide nutrients for the life I was growing, and stayed away from ones that could harbor listeria and high mercury levels. I stopped drinking. I stopped taking my migraine pills. I held my breath when I was walking behind a smoker or when a semi-truck puffed a black plume in front of us on the highway. But I got caught up with trouble anyway. And I panicked. I swam against the current. Swimming back to the safety of the shore was more impossible. I could never return to how I was before this pregnancy. My blissful ignorance was gone. I tried a new tactic, and what experts like Dr. Jamie MacMahon, a rip current expert at the Naval Postgraduate School, suggested: go *with* the current. Accept what has happened. Ride it out. Concede to the power of something far greater than myself.

I listened to what our genetic counselor had to say. She talked about our options, she said, *If it is genetic, it is recessive. That means only a twenty-five percent chance of seeing this again.*

I nodded.

I conceded to Sophia's death.

And then to a second, and then third, loss.

...

Trisomy 18, also known as Edwards Syndrome, is a rare condition that occurs in less than twenty thousand children born each year. According to the Mayo Clinic, children present with hands clenched in fists, abnormally shaped heads, and low birth weight. At the sixteen-week ultrasound, our fourth baby, Evelyn's, hands weren't clenched, but they angled downward. Her fingers touched the insides of her wrists. Two weeks before, we had seen her hand clearly pointed up. We watched her skeletal arm move, swim through the fluid, wave across the screen.

Later when I showed my mom the ultrasound picture the technician printed off, she said, "She's holding up four fingers because she knows she's four months old!"

I had noticed the omission of her thumb while I was on the exam table. *It's probably just comfortable for her today to hold her thumb down*, I had thought.

"Yep," I said to my mom. "She's doing math already. She must be smart!" But not until my mom brought it up did I consider that her hand positioning might be strange.

Now, in this sixteenth week, her whole hand was down. *Both* hands were down. Her fingers no longer dangled in the clear fluid surrounding her body. No finger wiggled, neither palm raised up. All was static.

The high-risk doctor suspected it was Trisomy 18. Dr. Denney had done his residency at UW-Madison; he was a fellow badger. He reminded me of my undergraduate days in Wisconsin, of my childhood growing up in the snow and the ice, even though I hated both. He could have been my touch of home while I was a transplanted southerner in North Carolina. I wanted to like him.

His demeanor never changed from the flatness that entered the room. Not when he told us that her hands were abnormally angled and weren't moving (yes, we already knew), not when he told us that he was concerned that there was overall low fetal movement (again, we knew), not when he said he wanted to see us again the next week to check on her progress (or lack thereof).

When he suggested an innovative new blood test designed to check the fetus's cells floating in my bloodstream for Trisomy 18, it sounded too good to be true. And it was. The false positive rate was high. Just as with every other prenatal test, it was designed to catch as many positive cases as possible at the detriment of casting a net too wide. If more people than necessary receive the positive result (meaning the test is sensitive), then at least most of those who truly have a positive case will know. And for those who actually don't have the disorder but whose test got swept up into the net, they are the consolation for making a test so sensitive.

That means the false negative chance is low, explained Dr. Denney.

When my result came back negative, I learned that Dr. Denney was a specialist without all the answers. He later made guesses at other problems my baby had: two holes in her heart, fluid around her heart, a triangular shape in her brain that should have been more rectangular. I may not have had the medical training he did, but I was the one carrying this child. *I* felt her move, kick, turn, and have hiccups. I grew in size with her. I ate what she should eat. I exercised for her. I was her home. And it was my instinct that I could trust.

I *didn't* have all the things.

THINGS THEY DON'T TEACH YOU

The following are things I didn't learn during my birthing class:

1. How you should consider taking the birthing class well before your ninth month of pregnancy "just in case."
2. How ~~some~~ *a significant* number of pregnancies (1 in 4) fail.
3. How to handle it when *your* pregnancy fails.
4. How to handle a new pregnancy after that failure.
5. How to handle a new pregnancy after a second failure.
6. How to handle a pregnancy after three failures.
7. How to handle the anxiety that comes with the fear of losing a fourth pregnancy.
8. How to have a miscarriage at home, on your toilet: a.) catch the fetus in a plastic "hat," b.) put it in a sterile bottle, and c.) drive it to the doctor's office in a paper lunch sack.
9. How not to cry at work when the nurse calls with the test results on that fetus and lets it slip that it would have been your son.
10. How to emotionally proceed with a pregnancy when it surpasses the longest one you've ever had (at twenty weeks).
11. How to throw a baby shower for your sister six months after you lost your own baby.
12. How to pretend you are happy to be pregnant when really it terrifies you.
13. How to calm a racing heart when the ultrasound room goes dark, or how to make your hands stop sweating as the cool gel covers

your belly, or how to stop holding your breath until there is movement on the screen.
14. How to dam the tears so they don't trail down your temple and onto the paper sheet beneath you.
15. How to love a child that you are afraid of.
16. How to stay positive when the doctor says your baby isn't moving, her wrists are bent unnaturally, and it appears she has clubbed feet.
17. How to call or text your parents and give them weekly updates on this bad news.
18. How to tell your boss you have to miss work *again* because the results of the ultrasound showed *another* physical abnormality and you can't stop crying on your couch.
19. How to accept the news when the test result for Trisomy 13 and 18 comes back normal, yet your child clearly has serious issues.
20. How to handle facing the imminent death of a child.
21. How to handle facing your own possible death.
22. How to remain happy for those friends and family members around you who are experiencing normal pregnancies when yours is full of troubles.
23. How to tell if you are going into early labor, and if so, how many medical interventions need to happen to keep your baby alive.
24. How to call or text your parents and tell them you are having the baby and, yes, it's two months early.
25. How a neonatal intensive care unit (NICU) will be necessary for the child born two months premature, when her lungs cannot yet breathe, when her mouth cannot yet suck, when her eye cannot yet open—and also, what the hell is a NICU?
26. How a C-section incision, the eight-inch slit through your lower abdomen skin and uterine wall, the one that allows your child to meet the world, allows her to live, will also make it nearly impossible to sit for eight-plus hours a day next to your baby's incubator.

27. How to find the strength to fight through the slicing belly pain to come to the NICU every day anyway and how pushing a pillow to your stomach to support your stitched suture will provide modest comfort.
28. How the blood loss from the urgent C-section will lead to an iron deficiency, which will lead to iron pills, which will lead to the worst constipation of your life (so much so it will cause you to miss a day of going to your baby in the NICU), which will also lead to an embarrassingly clogged toilet that your husband will take on like the beast that it will be (an incident of which he promises to never speak about again, and for the most part, he doesn't).
29. How the scariest thing about an urgent C-section isn't the four-inch long needle that goes into your back, nor how they shave your pubic area to get at the skin, nor feeling half your body go completely numb, nor the large hole they create in your stomach and internal organs, but rather it's the fear that your child will die before she is in your arms and they had forgotten to call your husband back in the operating room to hold your hand.
30. How when your premature child first hits the cold air and lets out the smallest of cries, your heart will burst with the confusing mix of fear and joy.
31. How when your daughter's tiny fingers wrap around your husband's index finger, you know everything will be okay.
32. How successful pregnancies *do* happen after recurrent pregnancy loss.
33. How the struggle to find your place in life—one that includes a daughter who died, two early miscarriages, and another daughter who fights disabilities—will roll into your identity as a human being and how you won't know yourself anymore without it.
34. How your empathy and compassion for everything that lives will heighten and make you cry at YouTube videos that include

children, dogs, kittens, and sloths that almost die while crossing the street.
35. How grief never really goes away, and will likely appear at the most inopportune of moments, like when a friend announces she's pregnant.
36. How you have a responsibility to share with your surviving daughter the sibling(s) she has or how to explain that the heart-shaped metal "toy" on your dresser is actually an urn and carries her sister.
37. How your appreciation for having everything in your life will amplify after you see firsthand how easily things can be taken away.
38. How quickly good things can become bad things, and how (over time) bad things can be turned into good things.
39. How there are many others who share this journey privately but would never share publicly (even if they long to).
40. How by sharing your own story through a blog, an essay, a novel, a parenting website article, or message board, you can help others grieve.
41. How *you* can grieve.
42. How you can live.
43. How you can thrive.

THE QUESTION OF RELIGION

Jason and I were studying abroad in Spain when we met, and while we both lived in the same city for the entire year, his apartment was far from mine. Madrid was a sprawling city, almost a country of its own. Metro lines—the orange line, the red line, the green line, the blue line—crossed like a maze of mole hills underground. The bullet-like trains carried us to and from the Universidad Complutense that we attended; to and from various *barrios* that had narrow bars with *jamón serrano* hanging from the ceilings, *tapas* of green olives and thinly sliced triangles of Manchego cheese; to and from the tourist spots like Plaza del Sol where Spaniards and tourists celebrated New Year's Eve by eating twelve grapes at midnight, and back to the innermost part of the city where I lived (next to the *Palacio Real*), to the outskirts of town where Jason lived.

One night we waited on the metro platform together. It was 2:00 a.m. Few people remained on either side, all of us hoping to catch one of the last trains of the night going in either direction. A small black child sat on his mother's lap across the tracks from us. His cherubic face made me smile. I don't know if he saw me, but I like to think he smiled back.

"I always wanted to have kids," Jason said. "I was twelve when my sister Jessica was born, so I have helped out a lot with her."

We had been talking about our families, how our own plans mirrored what we knew growing up: the marriage we'd want (full of love and fairness), the number of kids we'd want (three or two because...*siblings*), the way to raise the most moral of children (with religion or without). We agreed on most.

Still in college, still embodying the spirit of freedom, I wanted to travel, to hang out with friends, to see new places, find a job that would become my next identity. I hadn't had time to consider children. But Jason clearly had.

I nodded.

"I want my children to be raised Christian," he said.

My smile dampened. I didn't know if I should smile politely to this guy with whom I had talked nearly nonstop and laughed with over his silly jokes and his funny dancing with fists and hip shakes, or should I confess that religion was not a part of my world, my view, my opinion on how to properly create morals in another human being.

We'd work it out...eventually, I thought.

I learned that Jason had grown up in various denominations of Christianity—Mennonite, Brethren in Christ (a Mennonite offshoot), Presbyterian, and non-denominational—and had developed an interest in learning about other religions. I wasn't against Christians. Or Muslims, or Jews, or Mennonites, or Jason, his parents, or his devout grandparents (both maternal and paternal). I hadn't been raised with a religion, which made it hard to have much of an opinion at all. I often considered this an asset in a world already saturated in opinions. It left me open to meet people without thinking *I wonder what religion they practice?*

When our train finally came that night in Madrid, we boarded. We had left the conversation of raising children on the platform waiting for us to return. The train door closed behind us. The topic had to wait nine years before we spoke of it seriously again. Nine years was a long time to meander through life. It was time to finish college and move, unwed, into our Baltimore apartment together, to the objections of Jason's parents and his Aunt Bonnie. It was time for me to complete graduate school in clinical psychology at Loyola University before we moved to Milwaukee for Jason to pursue his graduate school dreams. It was time for my parents to get to learn who Jason was. For my sister to laugh when he made a mistake stomping on a dog treat on the carpet thinking it was a bug. It was time for us to get married, to travel to Disney World and Las Vegas and New Orleans. It was time for me to understand that his family was deeply rooted in Christianity, that Jason was raised to only listen to Christian musicians like Amy Grant, DC Talk, Michael W. Smith, and Carman, that his aunt would leave us a note on our kitchen table in that Baltimore apartment the day after our wedding *praying that we find a church to belong to.* It was time for Jason to realize that I was just as good a person as he was despite my religion-less upbringing.

It was time for him to ask me: *How did your parents teach you how to respect others? How did your parents teach you how to follow rules? How did your parents make sure you and Sarah were safe and happy and well cared for?*

It was time for me to respond: *Being a good person isn't about religion. We can have rules about respecting others, too. Religion is one tool to get those ideas across, but so is just modeling good behaviors and offering proper boundaries.*

It was time for me to feel Jason's angst when he stated, "I don't like everything the church does, and they really messed me up, but I don't know any other way." It was time for him to get used to the idea that there *was* another way. We learned together there are many other ways.

It was time for me to learn how to look inwardly to find happiness and let go of the fleeting world around me: the houseplants that browned and withered, the pets that died in my arms, of the babies I would later not be able to keep.

When we returned to the idea of children, Jason was finishing his doctorate work in mathematics. I was a psychometrist by then administering psychological assessments to children. We had bought our first home. We were different than the Jason and Laura that stood on the metro platform nine years earlier beginning our negotiations. And even then, our conversation didn't work out as planned.

DIARY[7]

5/7/2011
Sophia,

Tomorrow is Mother's Day so naturally, I have been thinking about you a lot today. I also found some old emails I got from your grandma about how excited she and your grandpa were to learn about your arrival to be. I saw the email she sent me soon after we lost you and read all the kind words she included from family and friends. Both emails made me cry. It is equally hard to remember the good things as it is to remember the not so good things. It makes me feel gullible to think that I thought all was well with you, especially after we passed the first trimester when most bad things are supposed to happen. I should have known something was wrong. I was your mother and I had no idea.

    I know celebrating tomorrow will be bittersweet. I will try to focus on how I love you and how I did all I could to help you. I tried to be a good mommy to you. I know deep down there was nothing I could do to save you, so by letting you go and stopping your suffering, I did the best I could.

    I love you, sweet baby.

---

[7] These diary entries were an attempt for me to get my feelings out during the first months after Sophia's death. They felt forced, contrived, and like I was talking to the thin air around me. I had never seriously kept a journal (only one as a small child in which I scrawled in my large handwriting how mad I was at my sister because of some dispute I don't remember). When my therapist, though, invited me to start writing in a journal because it might be *cathartic,* I did it. Because that's the kind of advice I paid her for.

LAURA GADDIS

...

6/01/2011
Dear Sophia,

Your daddy and I just took a little vacation to help us renew our spirits. I don't want you to think for one second that we have ever forgotten you. We will always be thinking about you and will do so for the rest of our lives. I love you so much, nothing will ever change that. I hope we have your blessing to try again and perhaps have a little brother or sister for you. I hope you won't think that we are just trying to replace you. We could never do that and wouldn't dream of trying to. You will always be close to your mommy and daddy, and your spirit will always fill our hearts. Please help us be successful in creating another beautiful baby—one that will not have to suffer as you did.

    Love you always,
    Mommy

CRITERIA I NEED TO MEET TO SELF-DIAGNOSE GAD (PART 2 OF 4)

Criterion 3[8]: The focus of anxiety and worry is not confined to features of an Axis I disorder (i.e. it's not due to other disorders such as panic attacks or social phobia).

I walked with my friend Kelli to Spanish class freshman year of college. Madison, Wisconsin had brutal winters. Snow, wind, ice sheets across the pavement.

I was terrified.

"Oh, god, Kelli is this whole sidewalk icy?" I asked.

"It looks like it, but it's okay," she said.

I stepped onto the walk. The ice was thin and fragile, but not fragile enough to crack and give my footing relief from sliding. My knees, locked. My thighs, tensed. Other students walked around me, their feet free to glide over the treacherous path as if there were no danger. Watching their easy gait wasn't enough to convince my legs to do the same.

"I don't know if I can do this." I said. Every muscle in my legs clenched. My kneecaps felt pulled in all directions.

---

[8] My fears, worries, and the limitations those cause in my life extend far beyond ice and slippery surfaces.

I stood in the middle of the path, afraid to step forward toward Van Hise Hall, afraid to step back toward Slichter Hall, afraid to step two feet to either the right or left onto the crunchy grass.

Kelli linked her arm with my elbow.

"Come with me, Laura."

She guided me to the back door of our dorm. The salted parking lot gave my legs permission to unlock.

"Go on without me," I said. "I just hope our professor understands."

I went upstairs and put my backpack on my bed. I laid out my coat, my scarf, and my mittens, with my hat on top. I sat at my computer and drafted an email to my professor explaining the fear that kept me from coming to his class.

WALKING THE RIVER OF GRIEF

> "No man ever steps in the same river twice, for it's not the same river and he's not the same man."
>
> — Heraclitus

The morning after I found out I was pregnant for the third time, I sat at the dining room table with the phone in my hands. It was ten minutes to eight, and I was convincing myself to call the OB/GYN. Our first baby, Sophia, had been born and died shortly thereafter only two years prior. The following year, we lost another pregnancy. By calling the doctor now, I was admitting that I was going to start the process over.

This pregnancy was supposed to span over the summer before we moved from Wisconsin to San Diego. My husband, Jason, had just accepted a year-long post-doctoral position at the University of California, San Diego to work with a senior mathematician in his field. It was a dream position, a stepping stone to land him his ultimate job in academia. San Diego sounded like a dream in itself. The sunny weather, the rainless days, the snowless winters, the beaches, the tacos and margaritas. This baby, if born at the right time, would be a California dream.

The dining room table in our ranch house was positioned right under a large picture window. I could see the neighbor's house twenty feet away. The birds, who normally sat on the fence between our house and Karen's, jumped down onto our gravel driveway. They pecked at whatever was beneath the stones. I wanted to be like them.

Carefree.

Searching.

Hoping to get something good.

Not afraid of what they may (or may not) find.

...

Judith was a therapist that Jason and I went to after our first child, Sophia's, death. She dressed in bohemian skirts, bangle bracelets, and fiery dyed-red hair. She once told us through her smoker's cough: *You cannot step in the same river twice.* I wasn't sure if she was a Buddhist, but her message—along with the garden Buddha statue that she was crouching near in her Facebook profile picture—made it clear where her beliefs laid.

Don't let the first pregnancy stop you from trying again. Just because it happened once doesn't mean it will happen again, she told us. Then she hacked; her face turned red. She grabbed the water bottle on the small round table next to her. As she gulped and gasped, I nodded, but I wasn't sure what to believe. It made sense but also seemed cliché.

But after hearing our sixty-something-year-old-crystal-wearing therapist talk about how nothing stays the same forever, about other universes where there might be other outcomes—the "quantum" (as she called it), and of synchronicity and how she believed things could happen just by chance and were not necessarily tied together, I was starting to want to believe it, too.

I didn't know of impermanence when I was pregnant the first time and my breasts hurt, my stomach was bloated, my sleep became turbulent, and my nausea peaked. These symptoms seemed constant, yet now I see they fluctuated. In the morning, my bloated stomach shrunk back to normal. The breast tenderness wore on and off. A bean burrito (no onion) and a Baja beef chalupa from Taco Bell sounded delicious for one meal and watermelon for the next. My body was in flux. Shifting. Changing. Malleable.

Once Sophia was born, my womb which had held a baby, let go of the life it once tried to grow. Here one day, gone the next.

After Sophia died, I wanted to reach Nirvana without realizing that's what it was called. I wanted to be in a place where I could be free of suffering. Free of the pain when I woke up each morning remembering that she was no longer living in my womb. Free of the crying that dampened the shoulder of Jason's t-shirts. Free of the grief that took over my every thought, making me believe that without my baby, my life would forever feel sad. Free of the torture of constantly expecting the same outcome, of being afraid to get pregnant again, of watching others having babies and not having to worry every minute of every day that it would be the last time the fetus's heart would beat.

To get there, I had to let go of thinking my situation was permanent.

I had to let go of believing the grief would never end.

I had to let go of clinging so tightly to the fading memories.

I had to let go of the moments I got to hold my dying first child.

I had to let go of expecting post child-loss insomnia to disappear every night.

I had to let go of the fear of ever trying again, of losing a child again, of having to feel the heartbreak again.

I had to step in the river and trust it was different.

A year after starting therapy sessions, Jason and I left her office after our last appointment. I no longer had Judith's bright red lipstick-stained mouth giving me wise words and ancient sayings. I would no longer sit next to the mini fridge in her waiting room that held water and orange juice for her clients. I would no longer have to sneak a miniature Twix from her candy dish next to the fridge (because I was too embarrassed to have her see me take the very candy left for clients.)

I asked Jason, "Do you think we're ready? I mean, do you think it's a good idea to stop seeing Judith?"

He held my hand. I loved feeling his fingers intertwined with mine. It reminded me that my life was also his. I was not the only one feeling this loss. Outside of us two, I saw others grieve as well. My parents cried while the nurse brought them back from seeing Sophia's body in the morgue. My sister brought chicken salad sandwiches to soothe us as we left the hospital, giving us what little she had to offer. But Jason and I were the only ones who had just lost the chance to parent this little girl.

"We have to at some point, babe. I think we're both in a good place."

He gave my hand a squeeze. This was something he did to signal to me that he was there, always. Or sometimes, when he wanted me to move, to follow him to a place that was difficult to go. Like to a quiet home where the swatches of nursery paint had been put away and the "Your Auntie Rocks" onesie my sister brought her niece was now tucked in the back corner of a drawer beneath a pile of my shirts.

Before we left our final visit with Judith, she asked, "Can you describe the tools you've learned? Let's talk about them."

I said, "Well, I think I know better how to handle the sad waves. I can take a moment to feel that sadness. Allow it in, I guess."

Judith nodded. "Yes, that's good." She wrote on her yellow legal pad.

I didn't know how to say anything else. I couldn't commit to having changed anything aside from momentary destructive thoughts. I wanted to believe that I could feel sad and not be afraid of it. It couldn't keep me under the bed covers forever, even if it felt that way. The tears would even dry, and my face would take on new expressions.

My grief would peak at my sister-in-law's baby shower and ebb when watching *The Big Bang Theory* snuggled with Jason on the couch.

I had learned techniques to make me feel better in the moment: how to take deep breaths when my heart started to rupture, how to slow the blood flow that tingled my fingertips and stop the thoughts that threatened to make me believe that the death of my baby could be my fault. I learned that I could feel sadness and joy at the same time. I could cry *and* smile. The grief would make me livid at friends on Facebook for having babies, yet happy for my sister and sister-in-law for having babies. I could feel like having my own child was hopeless, yet there was always still a chance. I cried when I read about children dying of cancer or about euthanizing unclaimed shelter animals.

What I really learned, but didn't realize yet, was more than just using my tools. Still, what I learned carried me through the next two years, even if I didn't know it yet.

We said our goodbyes to Judith. It was sad to leave the stranger who listened to our darkest story. I wanted to stay in the comfort of her brown couch, her stale smoke-smelling pillows. There was something about being here that let me leave my own world, even though all we did was talk about our pain. It was doing so in someone else's space.

The stairs creaked beneath our feet for the last time as we descended from the second floor office to the back door exit. I knew exactly where the pitch of each floorboard lived.

For the last year, I had feared leaving our late-night appointments as the parking lot was always deserted except for Judith's old silver Corolla lined with bumper stickers promoting peace and coexistence, and our own newer silver Corolla clean of any markings. Jason's six-foot frame walked me, for the last time, to our car. He opened the door for me. We drove out from behind the line of office buildings and out onto the wide, highly traveled Mayfair Road back to our small bit of home. The evening darkness drew us in as we exited to the back parking lot. Lights from the Mayfair shopping mall across the street shined a residual glow over the roof of the old square brick building.

We passed by Mo's Irish Pub, Caribou Coffee, Qdoba, Starbucks—all places we had frequented regularly. All had seen me pregnant and not. I thought, *nothing out here seems different. But should they be? Are they, too, in a state of impermanence?*

Am I?

...

Thinking about how Judith had told us not to fear trying for a baby again, it felt crazy. I felt crazy for wanting to try again, yet I felt crazy for not trying again. Each pregnancy ended in loss, but how would I know if one time it wouldn't?

I could now identify my persistent thoughts of permanency:

I'm going to lose this baby, too.
She'll have the same issues as Sophia.
She'll be born too early.
We weren't meant to have a baby.
Why do we keep trying?

...

The following year, Jason and I decided we were ready to try a second time. My spring pregnancy began in late February.

Then I had another miscarriage at nine weeks.

It ended in mid-April after waiting four weeks for the baby with a missing heartbeat to miscarry. This loss was different than the first. It ended before I could allow myself to become too attached. It happened at home, in our small bathroom with me crying over the toilet. It seemed to make my heart ache less. I felt more numb. More repelled by what my body just did. More determined to make a pregnancy work, despite the horrors of seeing my baby flush away.

I knew this would happen again, I thought.
I shouldn't have trusted in my body.
I shouldn't have trusted the Universe.
I never want to do this again.

Yet, I couldn't deny the differences. Sophia had been born alive and died in my husband's arms. Her body could sustain itself, just not long enough. Her limbs were malformed. Her heart, weak. Her body, two weeks behind the growth charts. Our spring baby never even had the chance to prove that it was a body capable of a beating heart. I didn't carry that baby long enough to know if its knees would be bent sideways or its wrists would be stuck bending downward. Perhaps that baby was a loss from chromosome abnormalities, something the amniocentesis proved wasn't true for Sophia.

Perhaps we could hit a time where the difference is the baby actually lives.

...

Then came my summer pregnancy. It was the third time in as many years. I called out to Jason. He left the home office where he was working on his graduate dissertation work.

He looked at the two pink lines and immediately hugged me. I cried into his T-shirt. I wanted to have a baby, but I didn't want to go through this again. The doctor's visits, the ultrasounds, the blood tests, the bad news about a deformity with the legs, or clubfeet, or a receding chin. Perhaps Jason didn't worry about those things. I didn't know as he never said it out loud. But he was always there by my side. He held my hand when the technicians warmed the gel, put the wands on my belly, and turned the screens away when there was trouble.

He never let go.

He sat with me as we had waited for the doctor to return with the technician when we first learned that Sophia wasn't going to make it. He smiled when a baby still had a heartbeat and wiped away a quick tear when he knew the baby's heart had stopped before I could even see the screen. When I was in the emergency room once with the spring baby after a bad bleed, he smiled and squeezed my hand as he watched the screen. I knew what he was seeing even when the technician was silent. His hope gave me my hope.

He held my hand as we sat on the couch after the spring baby disappeared from our lives.

And now he held me as we had a third chance.

"What if it happens again?" I asked Jason.

"I dunno. Maybe it won't," he said. His arms held me tight.

"Maybe. But maybe it *will*." I paused. He never let go. "I just keep thinking about what Judith told us."

He rubbed my back. He knew I liked soft touches along my spine.

"What was that?" he asked.

"We can't step in the same river twice. This time feels like it will be the same, though. But maybe that's because I don't know anything different. This time *could* be different. Do you think?"

"Yeah, I remember that. I dunno. I really don't. I think we just need to take this one day at a time."

I knew he was right. Taking one day at a time is what I did when we first learned of Sophia's issues, and then again when she was born and died. Each morning, I woke up, and reminded myself of where I was in this cycle. Was I pregnant? Was I not? Was I waiting for a miscarriage? If only I could know which day would be the one we lose another baby. I wondered if there was a way I could skip that day this time.

"I guess I have to call the doctor," I said, "Probably as soon as possible given what happened last time."

"Yeah, that might be a good idea, babe."

He finally let his arms fall off of my shoulders. The cold air took his place. He grabbed my hand and led me to the couch.

Jason suggested we watch something on TV, as if he knew I needed to forget what would come next, about the journey that had always led to disaster. I needed to watch a sitcom so I wouldn't cry in the hallway.

I wanted to call the doctor right then, but it was evening. If I could just call, get past the dialing, and ringing, and explaining, I could find my breath again. If I could just get a date down on my Google calendar and share it with Jason so both of our phones would be sure to *ding!* with a thirty-minute reminder the day of the appointment, then I could release the worry of forgetting.

Waiting until morning seemed impossible--what if I lost the baby that night? What if, just like before, I woke up with blood soaking my pajama pants and I hardly make it to the bathroom before the blood clot dislodges with a plop into the toilet water? What if a clot lodges itself again between the placenta and the uterine wall causing a placental abruption and cuts off the life-sustaining nutrients my baby needs? What if, once again, I'll have to be the mother who lets her child go while helplessly sitting on the bathroom floor?

The television show we turned on, whatever it might have been, was background to my thoughts. *What about when I do finally get through to the office in the morning and I make my way into the office for my first visit? Is there any way I can do this without actually going into the doctor? Without seeing all the wrong that is going on (I assume) with this baby that we have yet to meet? Is the ultrasound going to show us bent limbs and reduced fetal movement? Will the heart still be beating?*

When, that next morning, the clock finally showed eight, I knew the OB/GYN's office had opened. My fingers brought up the doctor's number in my contacts.

I took a deep breath.

I hit the green call button.

Outside, the birds still hopped along the stones. They followed each other to new spots that promised more grubs and worms. I rubbed my index finger along the grains in the wooden table. The birds began pecking in a new spot.

A woman's voice: "You've reached Aurora Women's Pavilion. Please listen carefully as our menu has changed. Press one if you want to schedule, cancel, or change an appointment…."

I hit one.

"Hello? Aurora Women's Pavilion OB/GYN. How may I help you?"

"Yes, hi…I think I'm pregnant…I had a positive test…and I have a history of miscarriage so I just thought I'd call early on….is there a way I can get in as soon as possible…"

The receptionist was clicking. Her breathing, heavy. "Let's see here," she said. "We can get you in next week."

"Yeah, okay, that sounds good." I didn't even look at my calendar. One of the birds outside had found a worm. It carried it back to the grass, hopped two steps, and flew back to the fence. It had found the nourishment it needed. What its babies needed.

The receptionist's voice had been chipper. She was unfazed by the loss I had endured. Yet, she was the gateway between me, my baby, and my hopeful protector.

When the appointment was set, I put the phone back down. The remaining birds outside continued pecking, still not finding whatever it was they wanted to find.

...

Judith had believed in letting go of permanence: of our loss, of our grief, of our story. Non-attachment to an event, even one as traumatic as child loss, could lead to enlightenment. It creates space to understand that nothing repeats, even when we perceive that it does. I wanted to believe Judith was right when she said we couldn't walk in the same river twice, even after on paper, two miscarriages seemed like the beginning of a pattern.

If I could have visited Judith again, two years after that last appointment, I would have answered her differently. I would say I now knew that grief was a journey. It would never—no matter how helpless I felt—leave me stranded in one place for too long.

And a slow incline to happiness was possible, even if the summer pregnancy was to end at twelve weeks, two months before we ever made it to San Diego.

Part 2: Tiling Pieces

TERMS I NEED TO UNDERSTAND

Anatomy Scan (aka Anomaly Scan, level 2 ultrasound): *a pregnancy ultrasound performed between 18–22 weeks of gestational age. The International Society of Ultrasound in Obstetrics and Gynecology (ISUOG) recommends that this ultrasound is performed as a matter of routine prenatal care. The function of the ultrasound is to measure the fetus so that growth abnormalities can be recognized quickly later in pregnancy, and to assess for congenital malformations and multiple pregnancies (i.e. twins).*[9]

Alpha-fetoprotein (aka AFP, α-fetoprotein, alpha-1-fetoprotein, alpha-fetoglobulin, *or alpha fetal protein):* *is measured in pregnant women through the analysis of maternal blood or amniotic fluid as a screening test for certain developmental abnormalities.*

---

[9] It was as this type of ultrasound that I had first learned what it meant to be carrying a child with anomalies. 'Anomalies' wasn't even a word I had remembered using before. It made me think of sea anemones, of creatures that were oddly shaped, bent at the arms and twisted at the legs, swimming endlessly in the saltwater looking for its food, its home. Sophia's legs had been bent at the knees. They folded inward at impossible angles. Our fourth child, Evelyn, was seen drinking her own amniotic fluid on the screen during her scan. "The fetus drinks their own fluid, then urinates it back into the amniotic fluid, and drinks it again. It's how they get their kidneys functioning," the MFM doctor said. It was the only normal function she appeared to have at the time.

During my fourth pregnancy, I continued working as usual at the neuropsychology office in North Carolina. I was sitting at my desk, scoring a patient's psychological evaluation, when the nurse called.

"Your alpha-fetoprotein came back elevated. That could mean your baby has something wrong, like spina bifida," she said.

Like most tests I had over the course of four pregnancies, the *could mean* she used to buffer her words carried a lot of weight. It could also be heard as: *could not*.

Bicornuate uterus (aka septated uterus): *(from the Latin cornū, meaning "horn"), is a type of Mullerian anomaly[10] in the human uterus, where there is a deep indentation at the fundus (top) of the uterus. A bicornuate uterus is an indication for increased surveillance of a pregnancy, though most people with a bicornuate uterus are able to have healthy pregnancies. People with a bicornuate uterus are at an increased risk of recurrent miscarriage, preterm birth, malpresentation, disruptions to fetal growth, premature rupture of membranes, placenta previa, retained placenta (which can lead to postpartum hemorrhage). In some cases, the nonpregnant horn can rupture during labor, necessitating emergency surgery.*

I didn't know I had a bicornuate uterus, or a septation hanging down the middle of my womb, until I was pregnant the first time. Even then, the technician, the doctors, no one could tell me what kind of deformity my uterus had. Was it 'two-horned' or just 'an orb with an extra skin down the middle?'

"We often don't see these kinds of abnormalities until during pregnancy and the uterus is stretched out more during an

---

[10] Structural anomalies that develop during embryonic development, so in this case, during my own embryonic development, my uterus decided to become heart-shaped instead of round. It is the only instance I can remember hating a heart.

ultrasound," Dr. Gariti, my first OB/GYN had told me. "Septations don't usually cause problems otherwise."

They don't cause problems unless you try to carry a baby. Even then, it may not have caused the miscarriage. If the fertilized egg attaches to the septation, that's bad. Nourishment is sparse on the thin membrane.

But Sophia hadn't attached there.

She died anyway.

ICE CREAM

My ice cream nearly dripped onto the table. I watched the white droplet slide down the side of the pile of soft serve that the McDonald's employee had semi-carefully crafted on top of the cone. The variety of handiwork I have seen at McDonald's varies widely—the industry standard doesn't seem to matter unless it means 'each worker shall do their own style of piling soft serve on a cone': tall peaks, short and squashed lumps, perfectly-swirled-spirals-towering-so-high-the-tip-looks-impossibly-impish.

Most times, my observant nature gets in the way of enjoying the frozen treat. Or the hamburger piled, too much, with an orange sauce and lettuce shreds. Or the French fries that were far too salty, not salty enough, or limp and paler than my own white flesh. But this time, my thoughts were not on the craftsmanship of the cone I held. Or of my husband, Jason's, across the table. It was on a vanilla drop that threatened to hit the table in what would be a silent crash. But it likely *would* make a noise. One that, if my ears had the sensitivity to capture the miniature sound waves that likely rippled from the table, I imagined they mimicked the rattling of the earth's crust as it splintered open during an earthquake. Or it was more of a pounding, such as that of a sudden afternoon drenching rain. The kind that allows raindrops to slam into windowpanes and tap dance with steel boots on the roof.

"You okay, babe?" My husband said. I forced my eyes to let the drop go. Of course, I knew I'd return to it as soon as I responded long enough to not be rude. We had, after all, just gotten news. It was news that brought us tepid joy. I searched for a glimmer of happiness, yet my mind flooded with scenes of horror from the past five years. These scenes often started out this way: full of promise but with a caveat. The news begged us to smile. To feel joy. We appeased this news's request by getting ice cream, just in case we didn't end up with anything else to celebrate.

"I'm fine. Just thinking," I said.

"It's going to be okay. We'll see the doctor as soon as possible."

His eyes searched my face for that note of happiness.

I looked at the empty booths around us. I wondered, *is this what I wanted? Why am I doing this again? Is this what Jason wants?*

The belt of my trench-coat-style winter jacket, the one that I had wanted to get for so long and finally purchased that winter, wrapped tightly around my midsection. It felt as if it were holding in what I was unable to maintain three times before. *Soon, this jacket may not fit me*, I thought. *It will be too tight to button or tie.* The fabric obeyed as I pushed the large black buttons through their slots. I loved the oversized hood that hid my face from the world. I was like a Jedi from Star Wars when I wore it. It kept me safe from outside forces. Or at least it felt that way.

For now, the jacket still fit as normal. I could only have been a few weeks along with this winter pregnancy. It was the fourth time my body allowed a baby to start.

"I hope so. I hope this time is different," I said.

Jason reached over and grabbed my free hand. I again attended to the vanilla drop that now threatened its dive overboard, sliding over the lip of the cone so slowly it was like The Blob sliding under the crack of a door.

When the drop fell to the table, spreading its whiteness into a pool, I was reminded of my third pregnancy when I ended up in the emergency room. I had been at home watching television when I felt something wet. It was a feeling that left me uneasy, even though I knew from reading countless pregnancy articles and from talking to friends that pregnancy does weird shit to a body. It can leave a woman feeling like a foreigner in her own skin: body parts expanding where they never had before, cravings for inedible things like soap, remixing of bodily fluid with the skin's walls so that some parts ballooned up while others shriveled.

By the third time around, I had known this feeling of wetness. It was an oozing, like my body needed to expel something so vile it pushed it out even when my brain screamed, "what the hell?"

I had run to the bathroom. The red pooled into the toilet bowl, my underwear had already been soaked. I grabbed toilet paper, hordes of it, wrapping it around my hand into a little bundle until I felt I had enough to clean up the crimson that flowed from my body. Lines of red dripped down my legs. Droplets fell to the white tiled floor. When I tried to stand, something dislodged from deep within my gut. I sat back down just in time to pass a palm-sized clot of blood and flesh. I was certain it was the baby. I had lost my second pregnancy not even a year prior, although the miscarriage seemed different then. But I couldn't explain otherwise what had just happened. When we got to the ER, the waiting room blurred. The triage room was bright, lighting me with fluorescent bulbs. I was a bug under a microscope. The nurse helped me into a gown. My own mental disturbance was protecting me from the devastating news again.

Yet, when I looked to my husband during the ultrasound, he had a slight smile on his face.

That's strange, I thought. *Why is he smiling?*

From my prone position, I couldn't see the screen, the white outline of my uterus, the baby inside, or the tiny fluttering of a heartbeat. I hadn't seen why Jason's eyes were lined with crinkles as he dampened a soft smile, or why he squeezed my hand in some version of Morse code.

When the technician left the room, Jason said, "there's still a heartbeat."

"Really?" I said. "How?"

"I dunno, babe. Let's see what they say."

When I followed up with my doctor, she said the baby was fine. She diagnosed me with subchorionic hematomas (SCH).

We had no way of knowing then, in the ER, or at the doctor later the next day, that our baby still wouldn't make it. Apparently, the expiration date on that pregnancy was set at twelve weeks.

When this softened vanilla ice cream now spread onto the table at McDonald's, and was followed by another drop, it reminded me of all that could go wrong. Eventually, the whole icy ball would be on the table in a melted mess. It would no longer exist and I would have to go on. But before I let that happen, I licked the side. The next drop that hovered over the edge was caught instead. I bit the cone. A jagged piece fell off and into my mouth, pausing for a moment on the fringe of my lip. Bite by bite, I finished the cone. The crunch was satisfying.

"Let's try and keep our hope going, okay?" Jason said. "I will if you will."

"Okay."

As we walked back into the chilly February air, I pulled the coat tie tighter. It hugged the seedling of a life that we again created. And I was determined to do everything I could to make this time work.

13-WEEK APPOINTMENT

I hadn't noticed the stain on my pants until I stopped in the restroom on my way out of the doctor's office. The wetness should have been an indication of what was happening. This was pregnancy number four, my winter pregnancy. I had survived many other gushes of fluid from pregnancies two and three, yet I tried to dismiss *this* gush as the gel used during the transvaginal ultrasound.

    I went into the largest stall, the one with the most white space on the tile floor, the painted metal walls, the porcelain bowl. I pulled my slacks down. I had chosen my blue work pants, ones that had enough give to fit around my burgeoning waist. They weren't my favorite. They were an odd color of blue. With a hint of gray, it was as if the fabric retained the bit of the misery from the February air outside. The color was a reminder that not everything in life dazzles like the sea, or the sky, or the blue that would be this baby's eyes.

    But that day, in that bathroom stall, with my long trench coat now untied, pants down to the floor, the red dripping was no longer contained within the fabric of my clothes. My underwear, soaked, sagged to my knees. Red smudges lined the inside of my thighs, my fingertips, my palms. I sat. And then stood. I was afraid I had left crimson smudges in places that other people would have to sit. I was afraid to grab the toilet paper with soiled hands. I was afraid to be in the bathroom too long. I was afraid I couldn't clean up the red tracks that now lined the rim of the toilet seat. I was afraid that the next clot was letting loose, right there, in the stall. I was afraid someone else would enter the restroom, go into the neighboring stall, glance down to the floor and see what looked like a crime scene in the beautifully white, sterile space.

I sat back down, unsure of what was going to happen next. There was no manual for subchorionic hematomas aside from my doctor's words: *Usually by twenty weeks the clots are completely reabsorbed into the body.* There was no signal when the next clot would decide to let go of its grip. And when it did become noticeable, I had no way of knowing how dangerously close it was to the placenta wall. When our first daughter, Sophia, was born, they found that I had suffered a placental abruption. A clot had lodged between the placenta and the uterine wall. It pried the life-sustaining organ from my body, and started Sophia's demise.

Would this baby suffer the same fate?

I begged my body not to.

I wanted control. I wanted my body to do as the doctor said, to resolve its self-created issues. Yet, this new pregnancy, at thirteen weeks, was feisty. It tried to show me it knew better than I did. It went against everything I wanted it to be.

With little recourse left in this stall—in this pregnancy—I cobbled together the best prayer a non-church goer could: "Oh, God, please let Dr. Wagner be right. Please tell my uterus to start absorbing the clots."

I grabbed the edge of the toilet paper, the industrial-sized roll that was housed safely within its plastic coffin, a place where it was protected from the urine splashes and E. coli germs that spread through the air with each toilet flush. But from this it could not escape.

I scrubbed the floor as best I could. It was as if I were trying to stop a bucket from leaking by cleaning the drops released from the underside. I wiped. And dripped. And wiped. And dripped. Meanwhile, my other hand held onto my pants, trying to keep them pulled up high enough to save them from the disastrous mess. It didn't matter anyway. My blue pants were soaked. It wouldn't make the laundry load any smaller if I could have saved the hems of my pants from the same fate. Yet, I didn't let go.

I wadded up more toilet paper and stuck it in my underwear. I grimaced as I pulled up my dirty clothes around me. It was all I had to wear. I tied the belt of my trench-coat style jacket close.

At least I have this, I thought. My heavy winter jacket had been too thick to be affected. The satin lining wicked away the blood trying to cling to the inside of the dark gray with squares, a pattern that could easily hide the misery that lay beneath.

Some of the blood had dried to the floor. I tried to wipe it off, scrubbing as the toilet paper tore to shreds. When it looked good enough, I left. Still, germs remained. DNA from my blood likely remained. If a crime scene detective came in with luminal and a black light, the stall would glow. But it was the best I could do.

Another woman walked into the bathroom. I passed her as I came out of the stall. She smiled slightly at me, the kind of smile one gives another when put together in tight quarters of an intimate place. I hoped I smiled back, but I was too worried about which stall she would pick. There were only two to choose from. As I turned the water on to wash my hands, the mirror reflected the other stall door swinging shut.

I should have warned her. I was relieved when I didn't have to.

...

This thirteen-week check-up wasn't meant to rile up the clots that begged to be knocked around. It wasn't even one of the extra appointments I was subjected to as a recurrent-pregnancy-loss person. It was a typical appointment. One that most expectant mothers go through. They wanted to check the nuchal cord thickness. It was an indicator of Down Syndrome (possibly) or other genetic conditions (possibly). None of their tests were ever "for sure." They always came with the caveat that they were not 100% accurate, and in many cases, presented a false-positive result. After we had lost Sophia, I wondered why we bothered to do these tests at all. *If something is wrong, it's wrong*, I thought to myself. *A test doesn't do anything but worry people.*

"The baby is too small to see with the transdermal ultrasound," the ultrasound technician said as I had been lying (again) on the exam table. "We'll have to use the transvaginal one instead."

I groaned. I hoped it wasn't audible, as I knew she was just doing her job.

"I hate this kind of ultrasound," I said to Jason. It was the kind that lit up the baby from the inside. It was invasive and knew just how to provoke blood clots.

"I know. It should be quick. I hope."

When the baby showed up on the screen, I held my breath. I forgot about the fact that I was no longer wearing pants or that this bodily intrusion may cause a war between my uterus and the clots. The summer baby's heartbeat stopped at twelve weeks. We had only made it past that once before with Sophia.

The technician pointed out the baby on the screen.

My neck craned up. With nothing but one flat, paper-covered pillow beneath my head, I had the worst view. The injustice intensified when the pain in my neck forced me to put my head back down.

Was it moving? I wanted to ask so badly of Jason or the technician, but the hushed tone in the room kept me from even breathing too loud. It felt as if the outcome of this ultrasound depended on me doing the right things: to not move, to not breathe the wrong air, to not let a tear fall, to not question things I may not want to know the answer to.

"The baby is moving all around," the technician said. I was relieved she knew to say what I was too afraid to ask. The air I had been so afraid to breathe, what I kept so shallow in my chest so as to not disturb my baby, escaped. It felt good to breathe. To take in the air like Jason was able to do, like the technician did all day. She likely had no idea how critical those words were. She said it as if she had ordered a vanilla ice cream cone after finishing her Big Mac. If I had said it, I would have screamed it like I had just won the Mega Millions.

Jason couldn't wrap me in his arms, or squeeze my shoulders. He couldn't kiss the top of my head or the back of my hand like he had done so many times since we first dated. But he could squeeze my fist. He kept squeezing until I relented and looked up at him. My hand wouldn't let go of his. I was afraid to feel love for a child who was still with us but may not be at any other moment.

This was the first time during a pregnancy that we saw our baby move. Sophia, even though she grew larger in her twenty weeks in my womb, hardly moved. At her anatomy scan, I had to get up and walk the halls, roll around on the table, and drink caffeinated soda to induce her to turn what the technician called "a bit." Even then, I never saw it for myself.

This baby, though. It waved its tiny arms and legs—just nubs but big enough to see. It pushed its feet against the uterine wall, bending its knees (its knees!).

When the ultrasound was done, I sat up. I put my blue pants back on. We waited for the doctor. It was a different doctor in the practice than I had seen previously. The only man. He had high ratings as an OB/GYN from women in the area, according to a local Greensboro, NC magazine.

"Nothing was found to be wrong," he had said. He carried with him an envelope. Inside, the technician had folded up a string of five pictures, all that showed our baby nugget. Included was a disc, the recording of the movement we had seen.

Stopping to make my next appointment, I smiled at the receptionist.

"When are we going to see you next, honey?" she asked. Her low-cut leopard print dress and red lipstick normally bothered me, yet today seemed charming. I would get to come back here. I would get to come back to the place where I saw my first baby move, where my baby bent her knees, where I left an appointment and was not in tears.

Yes, I thought, *when do I want to come back?*

"In two weeks," I said. It wasn't a matter of want, but of need. A label of recurrent pregnancy loss made me a candidate for extra appointments. Cervical checks for early labor were strongly encouraged.

"There ya go, honey. You have a good one." Sheila handed me the card. Her gum smacked as she said *honey.*

"Thanks."

Walking out was when the wetness began. Was it just the gel from the ultrasound? That's when I stopped in the bathroom to check.

...

The next day at work, the doctor's nurse called me. My alpha-fetoprotein was high, she told me. Her voice was robotic as she stumbled over the word "alpha-fetoprotein." Her keyboard clicked. She continued reciting her message, "It may be indicative of spina bifida."

It had only been a day since the ultrasound, the one that showed our baby kicking its legs and waving its arm buds. I had left happy, delighted. And now the nurse called to tell me the results of the blood test from that same visit might show problems.

The nuchal cord measurement was fine, but the blood test was elevated? I wondered. *Is that even possible?*

I couldn't make sense of what she said. Even in this fourth pregnancy, when I thought I had heard it all, I had no idea what she was talking about.

"Okay," I said to her. *Really, Laura? Okay?*

I hung up. My finger joints ached from gripping the phone.

I called Jason.

"What's up, babe?" he asked.

"I just heard from the nurse, and she said something about a protein being elevated. Something about spina bifida, maybe."

"What? I thought everything was good with the baby?"

"Yeah, me too. I dunno."

A tear fell down my cheek. I stood up to shut my office door.

"Okay, well, let's not assume anything yet. Let's just see."

The nurse had mentioned I would need to make an appointment with maternal fetal medicine. It was inevitable, going to MFM, as having so many losses made me high-risk. But I thought I would have a little more time before I would be subjected to the intrusive cervical checks, extra blood work, and weekly scheduling of appointments.

After hanging up the phone, it took me only a moment to jump on the Internet. Like a sweet tooth that could not be satiated by an after-dinner mint, I dipped into the unlimited chocolate fountain. It was a mosaic of fragmented pieces. Message boards, blog posts, news articles, editorials. Instead of making a clear image, the pattern it made was ugly, harsh, void of color. What I thought I knew changed, the fragmented pieces falling in different directions. What I thought I understood was wrong. On one site, it said that these tests produced a lot of false positives. More legit cases are caught that way, but it also "detects" issues that aren't there. Other sites described spina bifida—the way the skin doesn't close completely over the spine, the various levels of impairment it can incur, the odds of death.

How can this be? I thought. *How can we always possibly have all of the things?*

FUSION

At birth, I was deemed a healthy baby. I had both arms, both legs, all ten digits on my hands and feet. My weight, at eight pounds, was average. I probably cried when my skin hit the cold air, before my lungs knew they were pressing against ribs that were missing their bottom-most counterpart, a flaw that became detrimental. I suspect my APGAR score (a method to quickly summarize the health of newborn children against infant mortality) was within normal range. From all reports, I came home and joined my big sister just when I was supposed to.

When I was six, the pediatrician's physician's assistant asked me to lie down on the exam table.

"Something is not quite right with her spine," I had heard him say to my parents.

It was the 1980s, and physician's assistants were not common. Yet, this practice had one, and he was the first medical professional to take note of my deformity.

My spine started straight (presumably) as a baby, and gradually curved its way into an 'S.' When I first saw the pediatric orthopedic doctor, I didn't realize I would go back every six months until I had a spinal fusion in eighth grade.

My skeletal structure was genetically disfigured. I had an extra piece of triangular bone in my spine that had found the space of my missing rib. Pushing its way to the right side of my body, to a place a spine had no business going, was a slow-growing problem. It eventually threatened my ability to walk.

ᘮ

In 1984, Beverley Hyde, a social scientist, measured women's attitudes about pregnancy ultrasounds. In 1982, only ten percent of women received the scans. With its popularity, so rose the ambivalent attitudes and beliefs as recorded by Hyde: the mother feels happier and more confident, the mother likes confirming the baby before she can feel it, the mother likes to avoid the surprise of twins, the mother wants to share this experience with her husband. On the other side, women were anxious about finding fetal abnormalities (but noted that with the use of ultrasound, *we could cut down on the number of handicapped babies*). Women didn't feel the scan was revealing, suspected the ultrasound technicians deliberately hid information, acknowledged they couldn't tell what images were on the screen. Women worried that the scan wouldn't find the ailments that may be there anyway: mental health conditions, spina bifida. News reports at the time indicated that scans were not thought of as safe by some in the medical field. *Could cause cancer,* some women echoed.

In 1981, when I was born, my mother did not have an ultrasound. She was not subjected to the worries that the 1984 women (and the 1985, '86, '87, '88, '89....2015 women) were.

She did not have *my* worries: *What are they seeing? Why isn't the technician saying anything? Is something wrong? Will they miss something? Will they misdiagnose and cause my anxiety to skyrocket, disrupting my sleep and my appetite?*

It wasn't revealed to my mom ahead of time that I would be

born with a faulty bone structure. What could she have done had she known?

The women, when asked in 1984 what benefits having an ultrasound would offer, said *at least we know it's got all its arms and legs, everything it should have, and that's a relief.*

I wonder if naïveté would have saved me during my fourth pregnancy. *What did relief from witnessing a normal scan feel like? What if I could have gone into a scan hopeful, full of wonder, void of dread? What if I hadn't been told that her feet were clubbed? Or that her chin 'might be' receding? Or that her hands bent down unnaturally? How much mental anguish could I have been saved?*

ૂ

By the time I was 13, I had worn my Milwaukee back brace[11], a combination of leather and metals bars, a contraption designed specifically for my pre-adolescent body, for three years, twenty-three hours a day (exceptions made for gym class and showering). The guidance counselor met with me and my class to help prepare my fellow students for the change when they would see me—the metal ring around my neck and the three metal bars stretching out of my already oversized t-shirts. A girl, Lori, said *you're wearing a pajama shirt,* when I showed up to homeroom with a Garfield T-shirt, a large Odie on the front. I loved that purple shirt; it was long and one of the only shirts that fit over my brace. *No, it's not!* I said. *Yes, it is,* she

---

[11] There was no other option for my kind of scoliosis--the Boston back brace was easier to conceal under clothing and didn't have the neck ring. But that wasn't good for higher thoracic curvature, a curve in the middle spine. The Milwaukee back brace, designed in 1946, looked like a contraption designed in the Middle Ages. It took me a while to learn how to slide into the leather jaws, clamp the neck ring with screws, and pull the three straps tightly into the buckles. Impossible to hide, impossible to sleep in, impossible to wear comfortably. Reminiscent of a torture device, the metal ring around my neck often threatened to cut off my oxygen with a simple nod of my head.

replied. *I have the same one. It's a pajama shirt.* I despised her blue eye shadow and perfectly curled bangs that made one rounded wave upon her forehead. I walked away to find my spot on the bleachers, hiding the tear that started to fall.

This was a time when I also made some new friends, our town's three elementary schools now blended into a large mass of hormone-raged, socially inept, not-small-children-yet-not-anywhere-near-mature kids. Kristy, short and feisty and very much into Jesus, was my first new middle school friend. When I took my seat on the bleachers, it was always next to her. Her friends, Keri and Jenna, quickly allowed me into their circle, too. The three of them didn't care that I appeared half-bionic. They didn't care that the metal rim that ran around the circumference of my neck prevented my head from looking downward, from seeing my own feet, or the steps on a staircase; or that I had to remove my brace in the locker room, putting on display the Franksteinesque nature of my new body appendage. Ano, another friend I knew since fifth grade, had a gym locker right next to mine. She watched, and sometimes helped, as I shoved my brace into the narrow gym locker, straps always hanging out of the bottom.

By the time I reached eighth grade, the scoliosis had become unmanageable. Added to my condition was *kyphosis*, a twisting of the ribcage, and *lordosis*, an overarching of my lower back. Congenital scoliosis is a defect at birth. Something causes the spine to yield to an s-shape, and twist as it pulls the rib cage out of place. It causes a humpback. It was a feature that made me cry in the dressing room of JCPenney's when the zipper of a homecoming dress I loved wouldn't zip over my misshapen body.

"If the curvature of her spine progresses," my orthopedic doctor told my parents, "she runs the risk of severing her spinal cord and becoming paralyzed."

ɹ

Since I was six, I was prohibited from playing contact sports. No football. No gymnastics. No soccer. While my classmates ran around the elementary school gymnasium, I was often sitting on the side with the gym teacher. I was embarrassed for being singled out, for not being able to articulate quite why I wasn't allowed to play, too.

I was prohibited from ice skating and roller skating because a fall could jar my back. At a friend's birthday party at the roller rink, I sat on the side eating pizza and playing Pacman in the adjacent room. I rarely played video games, but when I did with friends, I was often eaten by the ghosts within seconds. The other kids squealed as they raced around the rink as Montell Jordan sang "This is How We Do It."

ɹ

Shortly before my inevitable back surgery, my family took a family trip to Disney World. I sat on the bench outside of Splash Mountain for the hour-and-a-half that it took my dad and sister to make it through the line. My doctor prohibited me from any ride that had large drops, loops, or spinning. Boatload after boatload of passengers screamed as they plummeted down the watery slope and splashed into the waiting pool. My mom volunteered to wait with me. She wasn't fond of rides (or water) anyway. We sat on a bench in the scorching Florida sun. My fair skin, pale like my Norwegian grandmother's, reddened quickly under the ultraviolet rays while my mom's tan Serbian skin, dark like *her* father's, appeared never changing. Yet, she made sure I put on my sunscreen. She tried to find shade for us to sit under.

My mom took me to buy ice cream—the Mickey Mouse-shaped chocolate-covered vanilla ice cream on a stick. The two of us sat and ate our ice creams as fast as we could so the white drips wouldn't have a chance to land on our hands, our fingers, our legs. She made those moments more bearable in the sweltering Florida sun. My mom and I didn't talk about the ride, about the gleeful screams, or about the fun that was denied to me, but Sarah was allowed to have. Instead, we complained of how long the line was and how we were happy to not have to wait in it. I enjoyed sitting with my mom; she tried to make my hour-and-a-half noteworthy, too.

When my sister came back, I asked, "How was it?" I was eager to know, what was inside the mountain? Was it cold when she got wet? How much did she get splashed?

She replied, "There were a bunch of animatronic animals farming. Briar rabbit and briar bear and stuff."

I hoped that someday I'd be able to smell the fake carrot patch myself.

༢

Trying to slow the progression of the curvature every day of each block of six months.

Going to the pediatric orthopedist,

MOSAIC

walking on my toes, bending forward in a
    barely closed hospital gown, lifting my feet up
and squatting *'like a baseball catcher'* every six
    months.

    Leaving school early when my dad
        came to pick me up in his short-
        sleeved dress shirt and   tie;
            he made room for me in his
            work schedule every six
    months.

    Fearing how bad, how curved, how pinched,
how distorted my body had become every six
months.

    Darkened rooms illuminating the glowing
crossbows of the machines, black and white film sliding in-
and-out, hearing *'hold your breath,'* every six months.

  Maybe that radiation still resides in my body.

ꙋ

Generally, X-rays are thought to be safe for the body. In low doses, the X-ray machines provide only .1 mSv (or millisievert) of radiation. It's the same amount that I would collect just walking around the earth for ten days. Multiplied by eight years twice a year, it seems it could be too much of what the medical field calls *'ionizing radiation,'* or the kind of radiation that changes cells. It seems like it could be enough to cause cancer, which the medical field claims is still rare at two-hundred twenty-eight in every one-thousand people. Ionizing radiation is more dangerous for children than adults as they have more growth to do and longer to live. When I later experienced four troubled pregnancies, and two of the babies had genetic anomalies, I couldn't help but wonder what all those ionizing radiation exposures had done.

ʟ

The surgery happened in two parts. First, they opened me up along my side, an incision running from the front of my right hip, over each fingered rib, ending under my shoulder blade. *This first surgery is to prepare the spine for the fusion next week,* Dr. Major, my surgeon, had said. When my parents inquired about getting the whole procedure done in one surgery, which would cut my hospital stay from two weeks to one, Dr. Major said, *doing the whole operation at one time would take a very long time and would be very hard for recovery.*

ʟ

After the first surgery, I overdosed on morphine. The hospital, St. Michael's, used a new method that allowed patients to control their own IV drip. Instead of hitting the red nurse button every time the pain became intolerable, I hit the gray button that laid on my bedside attached to the IV. It was supposedly foolproof, only allowing medicine to flow once every so often, set as a fixed ratio by medical staff. I could push it ten times, fifty times, one-hundred times in an hour, and only get one dose.

But when nurses change shifts, when nurses don't pay attention to the increases made by their predecessors, medicine distribution can go awry.

I fell asleep and didn't wake up.

My parents, sister, and grandmother were sitting in my room. When I finally opened my eyes, I didn't understand why they were smiling through grimaced faces. My grandmother, a woman raised through war-torn Germany, wiped away a tear.

"We thought we had lost you, Laura," my mom said. The nurses cleared away from my bedside. My mom and dad came up by the rails. Mom held my hand. I noticed my right arm tingled. It felt mutilated.

"What happened?" I asked.

"We don't know, exactly," Mom said. "You were resting and then we couldn't wake you up to eat. We called the nurse and she couldn't wake you either. Then they called a code blue and the room was filled with people trying to wake you up."

I thought I had just woken up from a deep sleep. *Is that what death feels like?*

"They tried taking blood from your arm but couldn't do it," my dad said. He sighed the heavy sigh he always did when it seemed he didn't know what else to say, or what else to do, yet had a lingering worry. "Then they were trying on your wrist."

My sister sat back in her chair with my grandmother. She was quiet. Her red letterman's jacket was still on, her letter for swimming stitched on carefully with my mother's sewing machine. I couldn't wait to swim with Sarah again. To get in the water, feel the coolness on my skin, smell the chlorine in my hair, kick the water away from me with each frog-legged movement. *How long until that happens?*

"We're just glad you woke up," Mom said.

ɹ

When the obstetrician told me during my first pregnancy that my uterus was misshapen, that it had an extra piece of skin that *should have gone away before birth as the fetus develops its organs,* I wondered if it was connected to my spinal deformities. Perhaps there was a gene, buried deep within my coiled strands of DNA, that mutated, distorted itself, and produced my *two* anomalies. One that created an absence of pieces in my body and gave me extra where it didn't belong.

What if I passed on my wavy blond hair, my blue eyes, my fair skin and scant dark freckles…and all the anomalies on to my babies, too?

ɹ

One week after the first surgery opened the right side of my torso, I was ready for the second surgery, the one that would expose the length of my spine to the cold operating room air and allow Dr. Major to finally fix me. This time the scar left behind would trail nearly the length of my back ending just above my tailbone. Bone fragments were extracted from my right hip through a small incision, a diagonal slit about three inches long; the bone chips filled in the cracks of my bent vertebrae. Dr. Major explained that with time, they would graft together. Wires married the metal rods to the bone structure. My spine straight, my rib cage twisted back into place, it was a vital procedure to continue doing the motions I was used to doing: to bend down and tie a shoe, to walk, to jump, to move my arms and hands and legs and feet. I was now supposed to be protected.

༄

The pain inhabited my body.

    I was in a stupor from the morphine drip.

From the *sutures* that now lined my side body, back, *and* hip. My *pain* pump was highly regulated; morphine no longer *flowed* freely.

The placebo effect of pushing the button once, twice, three times, four times an hour was failing.

I

couldn't

find

comfort.

༄

"I'm going to stay with her tonight," I heard my mom say to my dad once they stepped back from the bedrail. They had come to the hospital for the past six nights after work to sit with me, leaving only after I had picked at my baked chicken and Jell-O cup. They had a dog to take care of; my sister had school to get to. They were my grandmother's ride home. They had work to go to, dinners to cook, and the rest of their lives to tend to. In the week I had been in the hospital, I had spent every night alone.

"I just don't feel right leaving her alone tonight," she said.

ི

The couch as her bed,

nurses brought consolation—pillows, blankets.

Asked, *is there anything else you need?*

No, I'm fine, Mom said,

a smile forced.

Her face,

brave, strong, holding back tears.

Lying,

on my left,

the only side unscathed from a scalpel.

Her hand, her slender hand,

held mine,

threaded through the bed rails.

It hurts, Mom, I said.

I know, blueberry, take some deep breaths with me.

MOSAIC

My eyes, closed.

She inhaled.

I breathed in through my nose.

She exhaled.

I breathed out through my mouth.

Her tenderness held my hand

until I fell

asleep.

The last time the surgeon took a look at my sutures, the ones along my spine and the ones that twirled up my ribcage, he deemed I was ready to go home. I don't remember much, save the sliding of the chest drainage tube from under my right breast, a rubber hose that slipped between the ribs and carried out what didn't belong in the body cavity. The rubbery tube slid against the inside of my skin, along the bones, buried deeper than I thought. Or at least it felt that way. My mom held my hand until it was out.

Once dressed, the nurse brought my wheelchair. I don't remember how I got from lying to standing to sitting again, nor do I remember putting on the loose clothes my parents brought to delicately cover the fresh wounds, nor the ride down the hospital corridor, pushed by the nice nurse Loralie. My dad's van pulled up to the front door, each parent took an arm to lift me up and guide me (without bending!) into the reclined, pillowed, middle seat.

On the way home, I probably cried, from the pain of each bump in the road, from the twisting and turning of the on ramps and off ramps of the freeway. My mom slipped her hand around the back of the front passenger seat to reach for me, wherever she could touch, her light hand offering what little comfort it could.

I don't remember how I got inside the house, how my parents likely hefted me by each arm, giving my legs—weakened by two weeks of bedrest—the strength they didn't have to get up the garage step, down the hall, and into bed. My parents' bedroom, the only one on the first floor, was my refuge for the first few weeks of recovery. My first meal at home—not the baked chicken and Jell-O cup, but instead my mom's spaghetti—I ate sitting up at the dining room table, not from a reclined position. I stayed at the table for the ten minutes I could tolerate before the pain consumed me, before my parents led me back to bed.

I came home and joined my big sister, again, ready to regenerate the bone of my spine, to strengthen what my body wasn't born with, to be free of worry about the curvature worsening, of falling, of my vertebrae slipping from each other. To join my friends in gym class, this time without a back brace, without the limitation of the metal bars and rings.

I came home and rejoined my life.

FUSION (ACCORDING TO MY MOTHER)

CHARACTERS
MOM, 66
LAURA, 39
EVELYN, 5
DAD, 69

TIME

    The present, late morning.

    [*MOM is sitting on a barstool in her kitchen, LAURA is leaning against the kitchen island. DAD sits next to MOM. EVELYN sits next to DAD. DAD is helping EVELYN work on her Kindergarten workbook*]

    LAURA: So, I've been writing more essays, and you've been in a lot of them.

    MOM: Oh, boy. I hope it's something good about me!

    LAURA: Of course, Mom. I mean, not always good events; I'm writing about things that have influenced my journey toward motherhood, so you naturally come up as an influence. I wrote an essay about the time I had my back surgery. Do you remember when I wouldn't wake because something happened with the morphine?

    MOM: Of course I remember. It is something that will stay with me forever.... that will be hard for me to read.

LAURA: I know. It's hard to write. I just remember a night when I was in so much pain... and you stayed with me.

[*Tears form in LAURA'S bottom eyelids. LAURA'S face contorts as LAURA tries to save her neutral expression. MOM stands up and hugs LAURA. EVELYN sits at the kitchen counter five feet away*]

EVELYN: What's wrong?

LAURA: We're just talking about my writing, baby. It's just emotional. I'm okay.

[*MOM sits back down. LAURA finds composure*]

LAURA: When I wrote the essay, I debated whether or not I should ask you what happened. I decided I wanted to write it from my perspective first without being biased. But I'm curious if what I remember is what really happened. I mean, I was pretty out of it and I really don't remember much from that whole time.

I remember waking up and there were nurses all around. I thought you were trying to wake me up to eat and I just wouldn't wake up.

[*MOM shakes her head*]

No?

[*MOM shakes her head again, but stays silent*]

I remember seeing Grandma and Sarah (LAURA'S sister) sitting off to the side. I saw Grandma crying—she never cries so I thought that was strange. [*Pause*] So, what *did* happen?

MOM: [*Looks directly at LAURA*] Dad, Sarah, and Grandma had gone down to the cafeteria to get something to eat. You had just gotten out of the ICU and into a normal room, so we thought you were okay. We thought we were out of the woods. For some reason, I decided to stay with you. We were alone until a nurse came in. I didn't trust her. I don't know why, I don't know if she was trying to do something fishy...sometimes you hear about things like that, you know? Something just didn't seem right about what she was doing.

She was messing with your IV. I never got that sense from the other nurses, but something felt strange about her, so I watched what she was doing. She never said anything. She wasn't one of the nurses I particularly liked. I don't remember her name...younger lady, brown hair, a little heavier set....

[*MOM's face is solemn, still, serious*]

LAURA: [*shakes head*] I don't remember her.

MOM: Anyway, Dad, Sarah, and Grandma came back shortly after that nurse left. A couple minutes later, you breathed oddly. Like a gasping or gulping for air. It didn't sound right. Dad and I went over to you, and we tried waking you up.

[*Looks down at the newspaper sitting on the counter*] I could tell something wasn't right. You weren't responding. Your breathing kept sounding strange. I went out into the hall and found a nurse— a different nurse. One I liked. She was so nice.

LAURA: Was it Lauralie? I remember there being a Lauralie. I think because her name was so similar to mine, and because I remember one nurse being so kind. Short, curly brown hair?

MOM: Yeah, it could have been. I was so relieved I found a different nurse that I recognized. I said, 'Something's wrong with Laura' and she came running back to your room with me.

LAURA: Then what happened?

MOM: Well, she couldn't wake you up either.

LAURA: Were any alarms going off?

MOM: No, I don't remember any.

LAURA: That seems odd. Don't you think something would go off? Blood pressure? Heart rate? Something?

MOM: [*Shrugs*] You would think. When that nurse couldn't wake you up, she called for other nurses. Your bed was surrounded. Dad and I stepped back to give them room. Sarah was a mess. I could see how scared she was, how frightened. I took her out of the room and walked her a bit down the hall. She was only fourteen...still a kid. She couldn't bear seeing you like that. [*Face grimaces as if holding back tears. Looks despondent, deep in thought*]

That's when the nurses called me back into the room and asked me to go by your bedside. By then, there were doctors, too. Your room was full of people. They were trying to resuscitate you, but nothing they did was working.

LAURA: Do you remember what they were doing? CPR? Oxygen mask?

MOM: No, I don't. [*Pause*]. Your skin was blue. [*Touches her cheeks*] Your face was blue.

LAURA: Were they trying to take my blood? [*Flips arm over to expose right wrist. Traces lines where she remembers the needles poking.*] I remember something about them trying to get blood from my wrist.

MOM: Yes, they were. The nurses couldn't get it from your arm, so they tried your wrist. The doctor tried. No one could get blood. I guess it wasn't flowing enough. [*Pause. Audible breath*]

LAURA: Why were they trying to get blood?

MOM: I'm not exactly sure. I think it was something to check to see what was in your bloodstream, what might be causing this. [*Pauses. Appears to be thinking, conjuring a memory that was buried deep into the recesses of her past*] They called me back in and over to your bed. They told me to say your name. You weren't responding to them, but they thought you might respond better to me. To something familiar, a voice you knew. I was yelling your name, calling 'Laura! Laura!' Then I saw your eyelashes flutter and you opened your eyes. That moment will forever stick with me. I never felt such relief before.

[*MOM and LAURA tear up, again*]

LAURA: So, you stayed with me that night?

MOM: Yes. I didn't want to leave you after that episode.

LAURA: And that was after the first surgery? Not the second?

MOM: Correct. It was a couple nights after your first surgery.

LAURA: I really thought it was the second surgery. I thought it was when I was in so much pain again from the new stitches and having my medication restricted. I guess I was off with that one. Did they change my pain medication then? I thought they made it so the machine wouldn't give me the same dosage anymore... [*Trails off like a question*].

MOM: They took you off of morphine. They put you on Demerol, I think. Is that what it's called?

LAURA: Yeah, I think that's a pain medication, that sounds right. Did they ever find out what happened?

MOM: No, and at the time, I didn't think to pursue it. I was just focused on you and getting you well and home. Looking back on it, I wish we had asked more questions. Tried to figure out what exactly that nurse did with your IV.

LAURA: I understand, though. When Evelyn didn't wake up after her foot surgery, I didn't think to pursue anything with that either. Afterwards I thought about it, thought it was strange, wondered what exactly happened, but decided to focus on Evelyn. I always wondered, though, what happened with her anesthesia.

MOM: Yeah. There are similarities there.

For years afterward, you would joke about that time. You would ask me 'do you remember when I almost died...' and laugh, and I would tell you 'That's not funny, Laura!'

LAURA: I don't remember doing that, but it sounds like something I'd say. I don't think I ever realized how close to death I really was. I really just thought I was sleeping. All I knew was that you guys were all really upset that day in my hospital room.

MOM: I'll never forget it. Never forget how I had to call your name, the moment you opened your eyes. The relief.

[*MOM stands from stool and hugs LAURA. DAD and EVELYN finish the workbook page they had started. EVELYN closes the book.*]

THE END

ALL THE THINGS

Medical Progress Note (Mother)

Patient Name		
Laura Gaddis	**MEDICAL ISSUE**	**PROGRESS NOTES**
Date of Birth 06/19/1981	Pre-term Labor Risk	Needs weekly ultrasounds *(Will the sound waves from the machine disfigure my baby?)*
Patient ID ########	Blood Clotting Disorder	SCH *(again?)* MTHFR gene?[12]--Order test *(21 vials of blood!)*
Next Appointment Date Next week, then once every week after that, unless I deem she	Septated uterus	Could be a bicornuate uterus, can't tell from ultrasound picture *(What's the difference?)*; MRI with contrast needed to distinguish between the two *(Will*

---

[12] When there are mutations or variations in the *MTHFR* gene, it can lead to serious genetic disorders such as homocystinuria, anencephaly, spina bifida, and others. The MTHFR enzyme is critical for metabolizing one form of B vitamin, folate, into another. It cannot be a coincidence that the gene is shortened to MTHFR.

MOSAIC

needs twice-weekly appointments		*insurance cover that? Does it even matter?)*
		*MENTAL NOTE: should have done this **before** getting pregnant again.*
	RPL	*(How did I get here? Where does this go in the future? Are all of the medical tests, doctors' appointments, nights filled with insomnia caused by worries, doubts, fears, bleeding, and the obsession to feel my baby move going to be worth it?)*

Physician Signature:

Medical Progress Note (unborn child)

Patient Name	
NFN[13] Gaddis	**MEDICAL PROGRESS NOTES**

---

[13] NFN = "no first name." It denotes a baby who is a person, yet not quite. A living being that demands total assistance to live and thrive yet isn't ready for its own identifier. Still a part of the mother, it is referred to as such; my last name, identified

(Possibly 'Evelyn'? I've always liked the classic names. And 'Hope' for a middle name? I hope Jason likes Hope.)	**ISSUE**	
~~Date of Birth~~ **Due Date:** 9/13/2015	Increased Alpha-fetoprotein question of Spina Bifida	Schedule ultrasound with MFM *(so if not spina bifida, then something else? Doctor says "likely something else.")* *MENTAL NOTE: Stop Googling "Increased Alpha-fetoprotein."*
Patient ID ########	Trisomy 13? Multiple anomalies with limbs, possibly organs, fetal movement	Additional blood test, possible amniocentesis to chart chromosomes. *(Two of each chromosome is normal.)* *Deadly.*
Next Appointment Date Next week, then once every week	Trisomy 18? (see above for notes on anomalies)	See above. *Deadly.*

through me until she is born and joins a world that will finally acknowledge her. When I faced termination of our first pregnancy, this anonymity should have provided a shield from the angst. When I faced the ever-growing list of medical problems with Evelyn, it should have shielded me from the panic. Turns out, not identifying a baby by a name does not shield from anything.

after that, unless I deem she needs twice-weekly appointments		
	Hole in the bottom membrane of heart	*correction, **two** holes in the heart (Maybe.)*
	Brain region that should be rectangular appears more triangular	No additional tests necessary. Monitor future ultrasounds. *(What?!? MFM doctor seems to lack brain region knowledge and/or correct terminology for what he is talking about.) MENTAL NOTE: don't see this doctor again.*
	Reduced fetal movement	Continue weekly ultrasounds and monitor. *But she was moving more than Sophia ever did. Can a baby just stop moving like that?*
	Contracted wrists; bent 90 degrees downward	*Just like Sophia's wrists were found before she died. How does this just happen?*
	Clubbed feet	*Related to the wrists but didn't show up until the following week?*

		What will they find next week?
Physician		**Signature:**

...

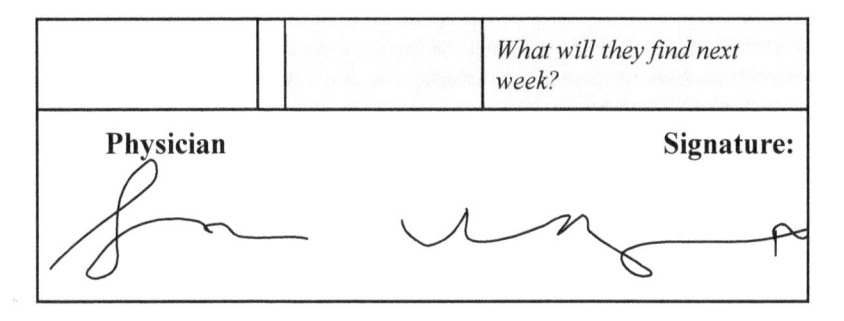

"You can't possibly have *all* the things," said Karen, the neuropsychologist I worked with during my winter pregnancy.

"I know, right?!" I said. When she had entered my office ten minutes earlier, she shut the door. She never shut the door before. My tears, the ones that waited for the suffocating space around me to be shared with someone, took note.

I didn't want anyone to see me cry. Karen sat in the armchair in the corner of my office. The chair meant for patients who came to us afraid of learning scary news about their memory fading. The chair meant for me to elevate my swollen pregnancy feet. The chair meant as a place to nap for ten minutes between patients when the hormones made it just impossible to keep my lids open. The chair meant to comfort away the pain that life brings, one way or another.

I chuckled. "All the things," I said.

I have *all the things*.

This baby has *all the things*.

We've always had all the things. With Sophia, with the spring pregnancy, with the summer pregnancy, and now with this one.

What would be the statistical odds of that? What were the odds that *I* was born with two deformities?

If I did have *all the things,* if I did defy every medical probability, ones that had me create children, yet not be able to keep them, I would be the world's most unlucky person. I would fail to have the good health I always thought I had. I would be a rare specimen, surely one of interest to scientists who want to study anomalies like me.

I couldn't *possibly* have *all* the Things.

WELL-MEANING PEOPLE

During my spring pregnancy, I went for a dental cleaning. I worried if a pregnant woman should even go to a dentist, but Google assured me it was okay. I had been just outside of the two-week-wait and took an at-home pregnancy test. I was nervous the days leading up to the appointment knowing that if I was pregnant, I'd have to say something. But it was very early, so there was a good chance I would get a false negative. The day I peed on the stick, it showed two pink lines.

"How do I tell them I'm pregnant?" I had asked Jason.

"Just let the hygienist know."

"Yeah, but *how*?"

"I dunno, babe. When she takes you back, just tell her."

"Yeah. I suppose."

I wasn't that excited, yet. I had a history. It was an awkward thing to tell someone I didn't really know. I could barely tell the people I did know.

But, the X-rays. Women get the raw end of the deal when it comes to radiology. Having to wear lead vests—the heavy, weighted body covers—to protect what we were naturally born with. Nature gives us a numbered amount of chances at producing life, and through a man-made invention, we can (maybe?) destroy that. We are born with one million eggs. By the time our bodies are ready to reproduce, we are down to three-hundred thousand. And, of course, we don't ovulate three-hundred thousand times, but rather three hundred. That's what is left of the one million. I considered the ways those three-hundred eggs are not all perfect. Irregular chromosomes, wrong genetic code, deletions, mutations. And with a man-made invention, we can continue changing what *should* have been into what *never* should have been. We can distort the DNA, the RNA, or the whole chromosomes that make each ovum. The very substance that codes our physical selves can be brutally corrupted. Or so we believe. There are reportedly no studies that indicate low doses of radiation have any effect on eggs, or sperm, or miscarriage. One study reported that the closer the egg was to ovulation, the more of an effect an X-ray done over the torso might have. Even then, that was in animals (not humans) and the scientists concluded that the risk of a spontaneous genetic problem was still more likely than an X-ray corrupted egg.

Had I thought about the timing of this appointment earlier, though, I could have searched the Internet for guidance. I could have made my best attempt at calming the nerves that sparked every time I was pregnant. What I would have found may have helped:

The possibility of an X-ray during pregnancy causing harm to your unborn child is very small.... Most X-ray exams—including those of the arms, legs, head, teeth or chest—won't expose your reproductive organs to radiation, and a leaded apron and collar can be worn to block any scattered radiation.

When I arrived, I did what I thought I had to do for the baby.

"Just so you know, I'm pregnant," I said to the hygienist.

"Oh, congrats!" she said. "I'll mark that in your chart."

...

By the next visit, six months later, the baby had been gone a couple months already. No more need to warn anyone.

I told the receptionist my name.

"Okay, Laura, you're all checked in."

The hygienist joined her now, looking over her shoulder to be sure I was the patient she was expecting. Patient privacy laws and all. HIPAA, you know.

"I see that you were pregnant last time you were here." She looked to my belly. "You must have had the baby?" The hygienist smiled that excited smile that people get when they see a fawn in their backyard.

"Uh, well. I actually lost the baby."

"Oh, I'm sorry to hear that," she said. Then she added, "Been there, done that." And she laughed.

Been there, done that. It's a phrase that denotes whatever happened was commonplace. Boring. Dull. Humdrum. Stale. Something that was not interesting to hear and probably not worth saying. Was my story one she had heard many times before, a story that every woman who walked into the dental clinic says *Guess what! I lost my baby!* to which she responds: *Been there, done that! Haha!*

According to Urban Dictionary, 'been there, done that' = *that is nothing new to me, tell me something different!*

It could also be a phrase used to imply that a person has experienced the same and understands. A sign of empathy. Had she, too, lost a baby? Or two? Or three? Maybe more? Had she, too, watched her premature baby die, naked and cold, covered in the only polka-dotted blanket she would ever have?

What about her laughter? Was she embarrassed to hear my news? Once, when I taught an introductory psychology course, I lectured about how laughter is often not associated with humor. We laugh at funerals. It helps us cope, releasing feel-good chemicals in our brains called endorphins. Perhaps she needed to feel better in the wake of my terrible news. Reportedly, women laugh more than men: 126% more. Maybe she just had a habit of laughing (a lot). Sometimes humor is mean-spirited, a gesture in response to someone's misfortune, or one's own good fortune over another. Laughter can be a defense mechanism. A way of trying to keep oneself from feeling a difficult emotion. It can be a response to a challenging or awkward situation.

I hoped she laughed because she wasn't sure what else to do. I hoped she didn't think she was more fortunate than me because she may never have experienced miscarriage. But even if she laughed out of awkwardness, I was the one who put her in that position. *My words were awkward.* All I wanted to do was be honest, tell a stranger (who had a lot to do with my medical health) about a medical thing that happened to me. I just wanted to be able to say difficult words that were now my truth and not make others squirm.

I felt the heat bleed over my face. I tensed my face to stifle the tears that started forming in the very inner corners of my eyes.

What I wanted her to say was: *I'm so sorry to hear this.*

Or: *Thanks for letting us know.*

Or: *You poor dear. I'll mark your chart right now so we never ask you about it and make you feel the horrendous grief and angst I'm sure you must have felt the day you learned her heartbeat stopped and her tiny fetus body slipped from your body.*

I nodded to her.

"Thanks," I said.

And I took a seat next to the fish tank.

I waited for my turn to be called back, to have my teeth cleaned, to have the X-rays and the dentist declare my teeth good, just like everyone else who sat with me.

SO CLICHÉ

1. Hang in there!

2. If it's meant to be it'll be.

3. God doesn't give us what we can't handle.

4. It was God's will.

5. God needed another angel.

6. You are young, you can always try again.

7. Maybe you can adopt?

8. Everything happens for a reason.

WHAT I NEEDED TO HEAR

1. I'm here to listen.

2. Life really sucks sometimes.

3. That sounds very difficult.

4. How are *you*?

5. We can just sit in silence if that's what you need.

6. I'm sorry this happened to you.

7. I'm here for you.

8. Tell me about her.

MESSAGE BOARD[14]

High-Risk Pregnancy Forum.

Subject: So many problems with baby ☹

| Mamawantsarainbow
member since Dec 2009

4/4/2015 12:05pm
⚑ Report ➥Reply | Hi other mommies/mommies-to-be! I am pregnant for the fourth time and am considered high-risk because of my previous three miscarriages. Actually, my first child was born alive, but then she died. Oh, and she weighed less than one pound at birth, so there was that too. Anyway, I'm now on my fourth pregnancy and it is so hard being pregnant again. The doctors say there is something wrong with the baby every week I go in (and I do go in at least once a week for an ultrasound). Has anyone else dealt with this? Am I the only one who thinks the doctors are trying to find things wrong with my baby? How often are they even right? |

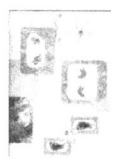

---

[14] Fictionalized yet based on personal experiences with discussion boards.

	1 angel daughter (born 20 weeks), 2 angels (April 2011@ 9 wks, June 2013@ 12wks)
	SCH, blood clotting risk, uterine abnormalities, pre-term labor risk

Re: So many problems with baby ☹

Soon2bemama2 member since December 2007 4/4/2015 12:10pm ⚑ Report ↪Reply	I had this happen to me too, but everything turned out fine! I don't have any answers for you, but I'll be praying for you. Just hang in there! 😊 👍 2 beautiful children: 1 boy (DOB 01/01/2008), 1 girl (DOB 4/27/2010)
Expecting_a_blessing member since October 2011 4/4/2015 12:14pm ⚑ Report ↪Reply	I have a large SCH...it was found at 15 weeks...am I going to lose this baby? Like, I want to be excited, but I'm so scared of what's gonna happen. Is that a bad way of thinking of this? I'm so sad all the time. 3 daughters (born 27 weeks, 30 weeks, and 40 weeks), 2 angels (DOB 6/19/2012, 9/27/2013) SCH, pre-eclampsia, pre-term labor risk

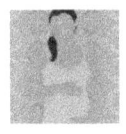

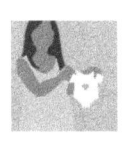

alwaysanaunt Member since March 2015 4/4/2015 1:31pm 🏴 Report ➡Reply	Hi! I'm new here, so pls be kind! I want like soooo badly to be a mom, but I've also had issues with miscarriages. I'm now in the 2ww[15] and hope this is it! Byyyyyyeeee! 0 children, 6 miscarriages, aunt to 2 wonderful nephews (DOB 6/19/2012, 9/27/2013)
mamawantsarainbow member since Dec 2009 4/4/2015 5:31pm 🏴 Report ➡Reply	Thanks everyone! It's nice to know that I'm not alone in this. It's still scary. Anyone have a good outcome despite all the bad doctor's reports? 1 angel daughter (born 20 weeks), 2 angels (April 2011@ 9 wks, June 2013@ 12wks)

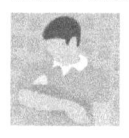

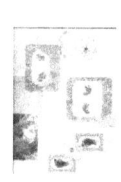

---

[15] 2ww = "two week wait." This is a notation often used on message boards to denote the time between when a woman thinks she may have conceived and when a pregnancy test will show a positive result. This is typically the two weeks after ovulation.

	SCH, blood clotting risk, uterine abnormalities, preterm labor risk
Mrspotter member since June 2014 4/4/2015 7:15pm ⚑ Report ↪Reply	Hi, mamawantsarainbow! It looks like you and I have similar stories...I also had three miscarriages and now am pregnant for the fourth time! We're essentially twinning! :) Anyway, I don't get all the bad news that you seem to be getting, but I am scared every day. The doctors thought my baby wasn't moving enough during my last ultrasound, and her growth is a bit behind. They are talking IUGR[16]. I'm just trying to stay busy and not worry too much. I know that's easier said than done!
fall_babysprout member since July 2014 4/4/2015 11:05pm ⚑ Report ↪Reply	I had a hematoma form at the end of my first trimester with my last baby. The best advice I got was bed rest, drink lots of water, no sex, and eat extra protein. My DD[17] was born just fine a few months later! Good luck XOXO

---

[16] IUGR = "intrauterine growth restriction." Refers to a condition in which an unborn baby is smaller than it should be because it is not growing at a normal rate inside the womb. Delayed growth puts the baby at risk of certain health problems during pregnancy, delivery, and after birth

[17] DD = "Darling Daughter"

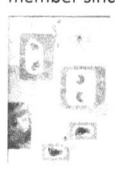

mamawantsarainbow member since Dec 2009 4/4/2015 11:07pm 🚩 Report ↪ Reply	Thanks, fall_babysprout, for telling your story. Funny coincidence—we call our little girl "baby sprout" too! I just hope I have the same outcome as you. Fingers crossed. 1 angel daughter (born 20 weeks), 2 angels (April 2011@ 9 wks, June 2013@ 12wks) SCH, blood clotting risk, uterine abnormalities, pre-term labor risk
kekethemomma member since April 2014 4/4/2015 11:50pm edited 11:53 🚩 Report ↪ Reply	mamawantsarainbow, you should probably just stick to what your doctor says, I mean how are we supposed to know any of this? Why ask strangers on the internet what their experiences are… some of us don't want to re-live that, and some of us don't want to share.
Mrspotter member since June 2014 4/4/2015 12:05am	kekethemomma--WTF? then why are you on here? Just to be mean? You can keep those comments to yourself. mamawantsarainbow--you have every right to ask your questions. If people don't want to share, they won't. And if they do, they will. ;) 🖤

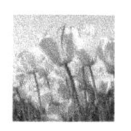

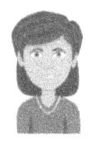

136

☐ Report ↪ Reply	
fall_babysprout member since July 2014 4/5/2015 8:00am ☐ Report ↪ Reply	Amen, sister! 🙏
alwaysanaunt Member since March 2015 4/5/2015 9:10am ☐ Report ↪ Reply	U C, this is the kinda BS i didn't want to deal with. Y can't y'all just be nice?
	0 children, 6 miscarriages, aunt to 3 wonderful nephews (DOB 6/19/2012, 9/27/2013)
Expecting_a_blessing member since October 2011 4/26/2015 4:13am	Is anyone still there? I know the last response was three weeks ago….I'm still waiting though….Can anyone give me advice? Please? See my post above. I'm really worried here and just need someone.

⚑ Report ➥ Reply	
	3 daughters (born 27 weeks, 30 weeks, and 40 weeks), 2 angels (DOB 6/19/2012, 9/27/2013) SCH, pre-eclampsia, pre-term labor risk

Moderator closed this thread 05/2015

DR. WALSH SAVED MY SANITY (AND PROVED WHAT I THOUGHT WAS RIGHT)

Jason and I sat in the waiting room at the pediatric cardiologist's office. Around us were chairs made of bright red, yellow, and blue fabrics, a table with marbles and gears, and the little plastic cars that a child can push over and around metal tracks. The walls were covered in paintings of trees, monkeys, and birds. I sat holding a hand to my belly. We had been referred to see Dr. Walsh five months into my winter pregnancy for a fetal echocardiogram. He was housed on the same campus as maternal-fetal medicine, aka the high-risk doctors, and the level four Neonatal Intensive Care Unit where my OB/GYN, Dr. Wagner, had told me I'd have to be when my daughter was finally born. Dr. Wagner's office was at a completely different hospital, one that took us beyond the thirty-minute drive back to our apartment in Kernersville and into the city of Greensboro, yet another twenty minutes up the road.

"If you give birth at my hospital, there is a good chance the baby would have to be transported by ambulance to Wake Forest Baptist anyway to be in the NICU. Then you'd be over here until you could be discharged, and your baby would be forty minutes away," she had said.

I thought about how it might feel for my baby to be whisked away from me, taken by nurses and doctors to be wiped clean of blood and vernix caseosa, the white coating that protected her from the amniotic fluid. I imagined how she might be transported; of course, that depended on what her condition was. Would she be breathing? Would her body hold enough warmth? Would she be bundled in blankets, placed on a gurney, face covered by a life-saving oxygen mask?

I wondered if I could handle it. Could I handle not having her near me if that meant I could give birth at the hospital I was supposed to be at (the hospital where babies and mothers whose lives were not in jeopardy could stay).

Maybe.

But then I wondered if Jason could handle it. The driving between my hospital and the baby's, relaying messages from the NICU to me over text, sitting at my bedside while the baby was fighting for a breath of air, going through McDonald's drive-thrus just to get a hamburger as he wouldn't dare to stop and sit to eat. I couldn't do that to him.

While the likely place of my baby's birth (and death?) would be at Wake Forest Baptist, where the high-risk doctors could rush from their offices upstairs to the NICU, Dr. Walsh's office was in a different building on the campus, separate from the hospital itself. It was a little cottage surrounded by the woods that edged the side of the property. When we arrived, it was late in the afternoon; there were few cars in the parking lot. Inside, it was just Jason, me, the receptionist behind her glass window, and the children's toys that our baby might never enjoy.

Our journey to this waiting room had spanned several months. I hadn't realized that there were specialists for pregnant women beyond the maternal-fetal medicine doctors. We had been peeling back layers of this onion since I learned of my pregnancy back in February. I hoped Dr. Walsh was going to be the core.

"I don't know if I want to do this," I said to Jason. He was next to me on the plastic-fabric bench. "I don't know if I want to hear that anything else is wrong with her. What does it matter at this point anyway? We can't do anything until she's born."

My fingers played with each other, first the left index finger rubbed the right.

"This is just too much stress," I said, barely shaking my head. "Too much."

My finger began feeling around the nail bed, tracing the cuticle that lined it, feeling the rough ridges that begged to be smoother. Eventually, my finger began pulling at this skin, wanting to make it go away. I tried to be gentle with my own skin; I tried to not create hangnails that would pull down the length of my fingernail and to the first finger joint. Pulling at the skin around my nails—often my toenails when available—gave my anxious mind something to focus on when I needed a mental break from whatever was going on. I needed a focal point (similar to a *Drishti* in my yoga practice) something to assist my balance when practicing eagle pose with one leg wrapped around the other, or dancer pose with one leg stretched out behind me.

Jason grabbed my hand, interrupting the sliver of skin from peeling back any further.

"Stop."

"Sorry." I let him wrap my hand in his. He didn't like how I picked at my skin. *You're mutilating your body*, he would often say. The warmth of his skin soothed mine. He rubbed his thumb over my knuckles. He often rubbed my hand this way when we were on a date at the movie theater. His caress moved over each knuckle mound, between them, from one side on my clenched fist to the other.

...

I was twenty-six weeks pregnant, the furthest along I had ever been. My belly burgeoned to a size unknown to me. At a visit to my OB/GYN, she had used her thin measuring tape to stretch from my pubic bone to the very top of the belly's skin where it met my ribs.

"You're measuring right on track," Dr. Wagner had said. "Your stomach measurement should match the number of weeks you are in the pregnancy."

That seemed like an odd way to measure what was working well with a pregnancy and what was not.[18] What if some women carry more belly fat to begin with? What if some had stronger ab muscles that kept their torsos taut? I had wondered how, if my measurement was so on target, was everything inside going wrong? How could the baby's wrists be static and bent, her feet curled into each other? How could her chin be too small and receded? How could her brain have a defect, one that makes *a rectangular part look more triangular*, as the high-risk doctor, Dr. Denney, asserted.

But, like a thread of hope that I clung to that everything could still be *okay*, the fundal measurement had been good.

...

By the time we made it to the cardiologist's waiting room, I had seen three or four of the doctors at my OB/GYN's office and three additional high-risk doctors. I had had weekly ultrasounds to check my cervical length and insure I wasn't going into preterm labor, to watch the baby's growth, monitor her limbs, and make sure her heart

---

[18] Things that can disrupt the accuracy of the fundal measurement: you have a larger body mass or fibroids. Other indications that a fundal measurement too large or too small could mean reduced fetal growth, a significantly larger than average baby, too much/too little amniotic fluid. My baby had none of these issues.

still had a beat. I had been told that her growth was on track by Dr. Wagner, only to hear from Dr. Denney that it was one week behind.

It was Dr. Denney who had drawn a crude image of my uterus on the back of a printed handout, a declaration of yet another thing gone wrong. It was he who decided the baby's brain was not right (even after Dr. Wagner had said it was looking fine). It was he who decided my baby likely had Trisomy 18, *judging off of my experience with anomalies like this*. It was he who insisted on the new-to-the-market Panorama blood test, developed by Natera, a company who based their worth in diagnosing genetic disorders. It was he who hoped he would finally support his hypotheses of what was wrong with my daughter. It was he who declared, when the DNA test came back with normal results, that there were still holes in her heart. It was he who had to be right about *something*, even when I didn't trust him to be.[19]

"There are at least one, if not two, severe defects. The fluid around the heart is particularly concerning," said Dr. Denney.

"The hole is right *there*." He punched the screen with his index finger, denoting the zoomed-in blurry image of her heart. "I want to see you back in one week to see if she is still with us." He concluded, "This constellation of problems is probably indicative of a genetic disorder. It is most likely what your other baby had."

---

[19] Despite Natera's press release (February 20, 2013—two years before my pregnancy) claiming to have "a sensitivity greater than 99% when detecting common chromosomal abnormalities…[and] demonstrated a specificity of 100% with no false positives for all the syndromes tested" I was informed that a positive result did not indicate certainty of the presence of a disorder. It meant there was a *chance* something existed. A false negative, while Natera declared unlikely, could occur if the "fetal fraction" or the fraction of the mother's blood that is from the fetus was on the lower end of the scale from 1-30%. How would I know where on that scale I fell? I wondered if it was worth confirming Dr. Denney's suspicions at the risk of also being falsely led to hope.

We dodged a diagnosis with the DNA test, but landed ourselves in the office of Dr. Walsh.

...

Once Dr. Walsh's technician placed the ultrasound wand on my belly, she barely gave me a glance me as her eyes locked on the screen.

"How are you doing today?" she asked.

The paper beneath me crinkled as I pulled my gray tank top over my belly. It was a shirt I had borrowed from my sister-in-law, and I didn't want to get gel on it. She would likely need it again.

"Uh, fine," I said.

Jason sat down in the chair next to me.

"That's good," she said.

I nodded.

"We'll be looking at your baby's heart today," she said.

"Yup," I said.

She shoved the edge of the paper sheet into the waistband of my shorts.

She turned the lights down. The glow from the screen was all that lit up her face.

"This might feel cold, but I tried to warm it up for you," she said. The gel squirted out of a plastic bottle that looked like it should have been holding ketchup.

"Okay," I said.

Small talk was normally something that caused me to want to shrivel up into my own skin. In learning how to overcome the anxiety of talking to people I don't know well, I once read in a self-help book that asking the other person questions could help. I had only one question for her, and I knew I wasn't supposed to ask it.

My technicians never revealed what they saw on the screen. Some identified the baby's body parts: the arms, legs, head, the facial features like nose, eyes, and mouth that opened and closed gently in the amniotic fluid. But never about what's good or bad.

"This shows the blood flow direction here," she pointed to reds and blues and oranges flashing on the screen.

"First I'll look at the blood flow in and out of the heart." She pushed a button and red streaked the screen. Another push, and it was blue.

"I'll check for the four chambers of the heart as well," she said.

She continued for an hour, describing how she was looking at the heart walls, the valves, the blood vessels leading to and from the heart, and the heart's pumping strength.

I wished vehemently that she was sending me signals for the words that she was not allowed to say.

Then she asked, "Have you thought about baby names yet?" Surely, she would not inquire about such a delicate topic if she felt our daughter would die.

...

My husband's and my legs touched as we crowded on the cardiologist's loveseat. Our hands clenched into a tightly woven fist. As our fingers interlaced, I dreamt of what I wanted to hear, yet feared what I had learned to expect.

When Dr. Walsh entered the room, his face carried an expression of ease. His words began as I clung to each one, looking for our response to Dr. Denney. I wanted to hear the triumph.

The cardiologist said, "I reviewed the imaging. We looked at all of the parts of the heart for how they are structured and also how things are functioning."

He made his way through the painstaking descriptions of each valve, ventricle, and chamber. With a final crude sketch on the back of a scrap of paper, he ultimately stated the most beautiful nine words I had ever heard: "I do not see any holes in her heart."

Dr. Walsh continued: "There is a small amount of fluid around her heart, but recent research has shown many children with this go on to be healthy. In my opinion, it is minimal and will not pose a problem."

This was the news I had wanted to hear for the past three months. It was the news that filled my dreams with images of my daughter dancing on the ultrasound screen, of my thoughts telling me that *this* time seemed different, seemed better. It was the news that allowed me to dream on, to hope for more growth, to know that her body would carry on even if her wrists, feet, shoulders, and knees needed help.

I waited for the "but." It was a word that always showed up. A caveat that often dared to dash our hope.

"Do you have any questions that I can answer?" Dr. Walsh asked.

He watched us. His face was still at ease. Maybe I was the most fortunate patient he had to talk to that day. Maybe I made the end of his workday better after having to scrutinize the scans of other high-risk echocardiograms. Maybe this last hour of his day was a bit calmer, before he went home to his wife, his children, his babies, the hour before he had to sit around a dinner table digesting his food along with the bad news he'd had to deliver that day.

Jason broke the silence. "Why would Dr. Denney think she had at least one, if not two, holes in her heart if you did not find anything?"

"The membrane that divides the heart in half can be very thin at the bottom. Sometimes the way the ultrasound is angled, it can look like the membrane is not there. I was sure to examine this thoroughly and we definitely saw it today. Whole and intact."

Whole and intact.

After all of the weeks of tests and appointments and doctors, I could call my parents and tell them something that wasn't modified with *maybe* or *it's likely that* or the doctors *think*.

I had never won anything big in my life—no large amounts of money from scratch offs, or Mega Millions tickets when the pot grew large, or games of bingo at my grandma's work picnics—but I imagined this was how it felt to win.

…

The afternoon sun filtered through the blinds of the secondary waiting room to Dr. Walsh's office. It invited us to leave, his business card in hand. I wasn't in a rush, though. I wanted to soak up the feeling I had then—a feeling that I hadn't ever felt, not since our first baby was conceived, not since her ultrasound showed anomalies incompatible with life, not since the second loss, the third, and during the entire winter pregnancy.

The relief.

The relief of knowing my baby was not dying in my womb.

The relief of knowing one of her major life-sustaining organs was just fine.

The relief of being able to let go of the thought that our baby would need immediate heart surgery if she were born alive.

The relief that one of the major symptoms of a life-threatening disorder that Dr. Denney appointed to our baby was, in fact, simply not true.

The chairs lined the perimeter of the waiting room, empty. With no one left to judge, hypothesize, and dissect this pregnancy, Jason and I stood in the middle and hugged. My cheek fell to the spot just below Jason's shoulder. It was the place my face always landed when we hugged. It was a soft hollow in his otherwise long, firm body. I allowed myself to lean into it. This time, my body had an awkward arch outward to accommodate my pregnant belly. We stayed that way until I had to pee.

The single-person bathroom in the waiting room had a large mirror over the sink. I looked at my tear-streaked face. My mascara had smudged. Flecks of black encircled the bottom edges of my eyelashes. I didn't care.

I was a normal pregnant woman. Sure, this baby still had issues with her joints and likely her muscles, but those wouldn't kill her.

As I walked out of the bathroom, Jason grabbed my hand. The baby was as it should be. My body was carrying a progressing pregnancy. Jason's hand took its place in mine. I looked back at the empty chairs. The waiting room was now filled with what I could afford to let go of. I left behind more than a few tear-soaked tissues.

Part 3: Art in Pieces

TERMS I NEED TO UNDERSTAND

Arthrogryposis Multiplex Congentia (aka AMC, arthrogryposis): describes congenital joint contracture in two or more areas of the body. It derives its name from Greek, literally meaning "curving of joints" (arthron, "joint"; grȳpōsis, late Latin form of late Greek grūpōsis, "hooking").

Children born with one or more joint contractures have abnormal fibrosis of the muscle tissue causing muscle shortening, and therefore are unable to perform active extension and flexion in the affected joint or joints.[20]

Both Sophia and my winter child, Evelyn, had the inability to extend several affected joints in utero. The year following Evelyn's birth I learned that there was an organization for AMC families, and a Canadian doctor, Dr. Judith Hall, who specialized in it. AMC is not a disorder, but rather a symptom of an underlying disorder. Evelyn's geneticist in the Wake Forest NICU, Dr. Tamison Jewett, could not detect any other physical features indicative of a genetic condition, yet she was intrigued enough by Evelyn's presentation, and that of

---

[20] Arthrogryposis was something my plethora of doctors were not familiar with. One OB at the practice proudly stated at an appointment that he looked it up in one of his medical books and seemed sure that Evelyn's tightened, bent posture was AMC. I wondered why a doctor's research and findings were remarkably the same as mine.

our first child, Sophia, that she asked permission to use pictures of Sophia, from shortly after her birth, as part of a presentation.

Dr. Edward Smith, a neurologist at Duke University, didn't feel that Evelyn was right for neurological treatment. AMC indicates there is an issue with the muscles, the nervous system, or both. "We don't know if the miscommunication between nerve and muscle is in the brain, in the muscle, or in the connection in between," Dr. Smith had said. He sent us off to a clinical study at Duke for undiagnosed genetic disorders. After six months of waiting, they called saying they found no match for Evelyn's condition. But as a side note, neither Jason nor I had genetic markers for heart disease or cancer (bonus information gained from having whole exome[21] sequencing done on all three of us...yay?).

With no answers from our own doctors, I watched a video that Dr. Hall recorded when she attended an AMC conference. I took away five things that no one could tell me while I was still pregnant:

There is often no identified reason for AMC.

There are hundreds of reasons AMC presents.

Drinking caffeinated beverages can help stimulate the fetus into moving more in utero, therefore forcing them to move their limbs so they don't develop the contractions in their wrists, knees, hips, feet, neck, etc.

Delivering a child earlier than forty weeks disables the restricted growing environment that keeps the fetus from moving.

AMC cannot get worse once the baby is born.

---

[21] Step one: take our blood. Step two: select only the part of the DNA that encodes proteins (which maes up only about 1% of the human genome). Step three: sequence the DNA. Step four: look for genetic variants that may have disrupted the proteins. Step five: find nothing. They'll hang onto the data for future testing (as there are always new genetic conditions identified). They will call again in six months and still say there is nothing.

I then surmised (with Evelyn snoring and drooling on my shoulder):

My continuation of drinking one fully caffeinated coffee a day was not a bad thing.

Going into labor two months early may have saved Evelyn from being more disabled.

I may never know the cause of her AMC, it wasn't my fault, and if we work hard enough she may be able to improve her physical abilities.

Club Foot: a deformity in which an infant's foot is turned inward, often so severely that the bottom of the foot faces sideways or even upward. Approximately one infant in every one-thousand live births will have clubfoot, making it one of the more common congenital (present at birth) foot deformities. Fewer than 200,000 cases per year are recorded.[22]

Ponseti Method: the non-surgical correction of clubfoot through manipulation, casting and bracing.

---

[22] Dr. Sheila Chandran, Evelyn's orthopedic doctor at Cincinnati Children's Hospital, treated Evelyn's case with extreme conservatism. She noted that Evelyn's case was atypical. When most children end their Ponseti shoes around age four, or at least by five, Evelyn was only downgraded to getting two of seven nights off a week from wearing the shoes by her fifth birthday. We cheered while sitting in the exam room. High-fived, even. But, without the shoes guarding her feet every night, I worried. I now watched her feet for signs of inward turning. I painted her toenails with a mani/pedi kit she got for her birthday, gently bending her feet upward, sideways, checking for the flexibility that needed to be there. Her contractures were resistant—the muscle tightening could overtake her arches, bend her toes into squished digits. Did I see things that were not there?

Dr. Ignacio Ponseti invented the method in the 1950s at the University of Iowa to correct deformities without invasive surgical procedures. As our first orthopedic doctor, Dr. Ravish, told us, it is considered the gold standard of club foot treatments.

It utilizes casting, a tenotomy (see below), and specialized brace shoes.

Tenotomy: the surgical cutting of a tendon, especially as a remedy for club foot.

When Evelyn was four months old, she had her tenotomy. Dr. Ravish had assured us it was necessary. Even after serial full leg casting, her tendons were tight. He couldn't stretch them any more and her feet would not walk flat.

"It is a day procedure," he said. He does this a lot, he told us. "It should be no problem," he said.

We sat in the small waiting room, a few chairs put to the side of a nurse's station, two sets of double doors blocking us from the operating room. Dr. Ravish visited us two, three, four times once the procedure was complete, each time saying let's give her another twenty minutes to wake up. We were finally led back to her room when he felt he couldn't stall any longer, or when he felt that having her mother and father bedside, talking to her, touching her, calling her name would be the key to waking her. We saw her lying, asleep, on the bed wrapped in thick blankets and placed under a heat lamp because her body temperature had dropped dangerously low.

"Wake up, baby," I said. I touched her cheek, her face the only exposed part of her body.

"It's Mommy," I said. "And Daddy's here, too."

"Hi, baby," said Jason. His beard couldn't hide the quiver in his lip or his voice.

For three hours we sat by her bed. I watched her face hoping to see her head shift to the side, to look at the ticking clock on the wall as it made the only sound in the room. Jason and I occasionally spoke, saying things like: What do you think happened to her? I hope she wakes up. Until our chatter turned more mundane: I just got an email from another student complaining about an exam grade; or, are you hungry? No, are you?

Occasionally I got up from my chair to check her face. Still flesh colored (with red hues from the heat lamp shining on her fair skin). Eyes, closed. Muscles just still.

Finally, Evelyn blinked open her eyes. Her long lashes batted. Her skin was cool under the back of my fingers as I caressed her cheek. I stood at her bedside, watching her small face poke out through the mummy-like wrapping that covered her hair, her neck, her shoulders, her torso, her legs.

"Hi, baby," I said. "I'm glad you're awake." I leaned in and smiled inches from her face.

"Hi, Evelyn," Jason said. "Daddy's here, too. We love you."

I wanted her to think I wasn't scared. I wanted her to feel like she woke up from the most restful nap of her short life, just as I had felt when I woke to a hospital room filled with medical staff after my spinal surgery. I wanted her to never know she almost died, not from her physical anomalies but from an error (gut feeling) from a doctor. I wanted her to never have to know the feeling my mother had, and now what I felt, when she thinks she's losing her daughter.

I KNEW

When the pain seared through my cervix, I knew what was happening. I knew she was coming. My winter baby, the one that made it closest to term, was coming. It was like lightning fired straight into the space between my legs, sending needles into my skin.

But that pain didn't stop me from denying it. I am too perceptive of a person.

I knew what was happening.

The evening before, I had been sitting on the couch, in my normal spot, watching Jeopardy and Wheel of Fortune, as had become my after-work-I'm-too-tired-for-anything-else activity. Stretching my legs out on the chase portion of our couch minimally helped my swollen feet. That's when she decided to move. Like *really* move. For weeks, she had become stationary, like Sophia had been. The bigger she got, the less she flailed her arms (her right one stopping altogether) and her knees locked in bent positions. Her feet stayed clubbed, but that was not a surprise. At each ultrasound visit, I wondered if clubbed feet could *un*club themselves. I prayed they would.

Now it felt like she had slid her head from where it had rested for the last several weeks to clear on the other side of my stomach. Judging by the pain that tore through my belly, I assumed she must have taken my extra uterus septation skin with her. It was the very uterine malformation that threatened the only home she knew.

I went to bed hoping to sleep it off.

When I woke up bleeding in the middle of the night, Jason called my OB/GYN. She asked him if I was having contractions. I told him I didn't know.

But I knew what was happening.

"She says we have to go to the hospital now," Jason said.

...

I put on my black yoga pants, the ones I wore when my baby Sophia was born, and when we left her behind. Inexpensive and bought on Old Navy's website, they were one of two maternity pants that I got when I was pregnant the first time. Those pants moved with me from Wisconsin to San Diego to North Carolina. I'm not sure why I held onto them. Maybe it was the memory attached. Maybe it was because of the price tag, and how they held up well. Or, somehow, I knew I could rely on them again four years later when I would carry her.

The ride to the hospital with the level-four NICU was thirty minutes from our apartment. Each bump shook my belly. Each mile felt like forever. But I knew every bump along the way. I knew the drive well from the weekly appointments I had to attend with the high-risk doctors. I knew how long it took, even when it felt longer. I knew how much difficult road lay ahead.

HOOSIER

When the orderly rushed into the emergency room to take me back and wheeled me down the hall, he said, "Congrats!"

I wondered why he said that.

When the nurse in the triage area took me alone to a room and asked me if I had been mistreated at all, I couldn't think beyond "no." My troubles were many but did not extend that way.

When she then allowed Jason into the room, him sitting in the only chair positioned in the corner furthest from the monitors, she attempted to give us privacy from the hallway with a pink translucent curtain pulled over the floor-to-ceiling windows.

When the nurse strapped the sonogram monitor onto my belly, the kind that wrapped around like a headband, she couldn't find the baby's heartbeat.

When I looked at Jason, his eyes were darting fast.

Once the nurse had tried almost every place on my belly where the heartbeat should have been, I thought: O*h no, not again.*

When she finally located the beating heart, and tried to cover up her incompetence by saying, *sometimes the heartbeat isn't where we'd think it is and we have to go to the opposite side to find it,* I cursed my body for not waiting until the due date in September when hospital staff weren't fresh recruits.

When the new ER resident doctor (two weeks in) came to do a cervical check, his eyes came back up from the sheet filled with fear.

When he said, *I have to go speak with my supervising physician and I'll be right back*, and he returned with the other doctor in tow, I wanted nothing more than to hold Jason's hand. Surrounded by too many medical professionals, he was as far away as if he had stayed in the waiting room.

When they told me they would try and keep her inside me as long as possible to give her lungs a chance to mature, I agreed to the two steroid shots.

When the nurse gave me a premade concoction in a brown plastic shot glass, telling me it had magnesium and things I can't remember in it, and saying it would help me in some way I didn't understand, I agreed to drink it.

When she also noted that it would taste rancid and salty, I held my breath and I downed the foul liquid.

When the taste wouldn't leave my mouth and I felt I might vomit, I practiced breathing out sharply through my nostrils as my orthodontist had taught me years ago when I gagged on having a mold made of my teeth.

When they said I wouldn't leave the hospital until she was born, I thought, *it's too early, baby sprout.*

When the NICU social worker came up and talked to Jason and me about how the baby will stay there after birth, I realized she might live.

When the social worker talked to us about how long of a stay we could anticipate, I wondered *What is a NICU?*

When the contractions started coming every few minutes, they brought in the anesthesiologist.

When Jason saw the anesthesiologist was wearing an Indiana University bandana, I saw him smile.

When he smiled, I thought of the time when we were first dating, and I went to visit him in Bloomington.

MOSAIC

When I thought of college, I remembered the time I visited Jason, spring of our senior year, for the Little 500 bike race. I remembered how we laughed in the sunshine and drank tie-dye long islands at the local college bar.

When the anesthesiologist told me that he'd be prepping me for the C-section, I remembered where I really was.

When he told me where he'd be sticking the needle in my back, I worried about my spinal fusion. *Are you going to be able to place the epidural,* I asked.

When he said, *I could also put you under a general anesthesia, if needed*, I cried. I didn't want to not be awake when she was born.

When they wheeled me to the operating room, Jason had to sit in a room across the hall *just until you are prepped for surgery*, the nurse told me.

When the fluorescent lights shined into my eyes, I focused harder on them to help me forget what was about to happen.

When the nurse sat me up on the side of the table so the anesthesiologist could place the needle, I stared at her scrubs.

When he got it on the first try, I was guided back down to the table.

When the blue sheet went up, the one that shielded my vision from watching her being extracted from my stomach, I asked the anesthesiologist *where's Jason?* The Indiana bandana was the only thing I could see.

When he called, *can someone get her husband back in here?* no one responded.

When the nurses by my feet rubbed cold, wet cotton on my legs and poked my skin with metal instruments, they asked, *can you feel that?*

When I said *no*, they said, *then we are ready to begin.*

When the anesthesiologist saw my face tighten, he left the room to get Jason for me.

When Jason arrived, minutes later she did, too.

When she was whisked away to the scale, we heard her release a tender cry. It was a sound we never heard with Sophia. It was one I wasn't certain we'd ever hear.

When the doctor was suturing my stomach, I turned my head to say to Jason, *they almost didn't get you in time,* and he said, *I always trust a guy who went to Indiana.*

SEEING EVELYN

Before taking Evelyn to the NICU, the nurse brought her up beside my face, just a tiny head peeking out of a plastic bag. The nurse explained that the bag was to keep Evelyn warm until she got to the NICU. Jason took out his phone, snapped a photo of Evelyn and me–her skin slimy and wet, my hair still matted in a hair net, and my eyes half-closed from a drugged exhaustion.

And then, with the hurried swarm of a medical beehive, Evelyn was taken away.

Jason hadn't left my side since we had been in the operating room. He had sat by my head during the surgery, only standing up for a brief moment when the anesthesiologist said that the baby was about to be born, and would Jason like to see? Once we heard the faint cry of a baby whose lungs were on their way to maturity, he sat back down, grabbed my hand, and said, *she's okay*. He talked to me while the doctors stitched up my uterus, my torn abdominal muscles, the skin that covered it all. He later told me this part of the surgery took the longest– longer than it took to open me up and pull Evelyn out.

When I was in the recovery room, a small three-quarter walled space that barely fit my bed and a chair, he planted himself and waited until I could leave.

I felt good. The pain that I expected hadn't shown up yet. We chatted with the nurse. We asked her when I could leave so we could see our baby. She picked up the phone off the wall and called down to the NICU, said a few "okays" and told us upon hanging up, *soon. We'll just keep you here a bit longer.* I had regained complete feeling in my legs, the pain was under control, and I was ready to see my baby. But the nurse never told us why we had to wait, if it was because of the inpatient work they do with all premature babies, or the long list of initial consultations with medical providers Evelyn endured, or if they just needed the hours to hook her up to the machines we'd later see. In my mind, something may have gone wrong. Did Evelyn stop breathing? Had her heart rate slowed too much? Maybe she was not thriving, even though the doctors in the operating room seemed so upbeat. I needed to see her. I felt naked without her in my body.

Jason straddled two worlds: his wife and his baby daughter. But the whole time, he never left my side. I assumed Jason carried the same worries as I did, but he didn't show it. Instead, he focused on my pain, asked if I was thirsty, and slipped behind the curtain into the busy recovery reception area to find the nurse when I demanded to know what was taking so long.

When the orderly finally arrived to take me out of the recovery room, Jason packed up my personal belongings: a bag that carried my phone, my shoes, and the clothes I had on my back.

The nurse wheeled me in my hospital bed straight to the NICU, before taking me to my own room. I barely remember any of it. I remember my bed garnering attention from the orderlies, other patients, and other patients' visitors on my trip down the hallway. People were staring, likely wondering what was wrong with me. Aside from the nurse, it was the two of us, just Jason and me, who navigated the halls, uncertain of what we'd find at the end.

The fluorescent lights blinded me as I lay face up on my transport. The NICU nurses clomped past in their crocs. Families disappeared behind curtains, the shower-curtain rings sliding over the metal poles that held up the only privacy each patient had. Hushed voices lingered in the air between the hanging fabric.

Monitors beeped. There was a steady hum that almost soothed the chaos.

I had never seen a baby that small, one born at barely three pounds with questionable function of her lungs, her heart, her eyes, her ears—all things that would be tested later in the NICU. In addition to her prematurity, we faced what the high-risk doctors told us was called arthrogryposis. No one knew *why* she had this condition. Arthrogryposis, after all, was the term for the presentation we saw on the ultrasound and now with her living body: bent wrists, clubfeet, low fetal movement, and knees locked into a flexed position. The joints, in utero, aren't moved around enough to avoid locking into unnatural positions. Low muscle tone is often to blame. There are hundreds of disorders that lead to this presentation.

I remember how big my bed felt next to Evelyn's—her isolette, a clear plastic box that covered her. Arm holes, two on each side of the box, allowed for nurses and doctors and parents to touch her. I couldn't reach her from my bed. I could barely see her as I leaned down trying to keep my sutures together.

I couldn't see her face. The CPAP mask was nearly as large as her head, her eyes, which had yet to open, were barely above the blue edge of the mask.

"Is she okay?" I asked. I wasn't sure who was around, the anesthesia and pain medication made my surroundings fuzzy. I was focusing only on the tiny baby in the box.

"I think she's going to be fine," said Jason, "At least that's what they said in the operating room before they took her down here."

When I saw Evelyn with the mask over her face, my stomach lurched. I strained to look closer.

"Why does she need the mask?" I asked.

The nurse responded, "Babies this small often have trouble breathing on their own. She was born before the steroids we gave you could have strengthened her underdeveloped lungs, so we do this as a precaution. She is doing well with it though."

I assumed that was a good thing. The steroid shot had only been administered a few hours before her urgent delivery. I couldn't hold onto the pregnancy long enough to get her the 24-hours the ER doctor had said was necessary to get the series of two shots and have the steroids reach Evelyn's lungs. Anything that the nurse told me that didn't sound urgent was, to me, a good thing.

"Why is she in the box? Can we hold her?" I asked.

The nurse walked to the other side of the isolette, putting her arms through the holes to reach inside. She covered Evelyn's naked body pulling the blanket as close to under her chin as she could.

"We'll see tomorrow if she can come out. She's in here because babies this small can't sustain their own body temperatures. If she does okay tonight, she could come out and be held for a little bit at a time before she gets too cold."

They could put some clothes on her! I thought. I didn't realize then that not only did we not have any preemie-sized clothing for her, but that even if we had the clothes, Evelyn would have been too small for them. The diaper was her only clothing, aside from the layers of blankets.

I was only allowed to stay a few minutes before the orderly took me to my room. I probably fell asleep quickly, a combination of the sedative medication, the pain that was beginning to emerge, the exhaustion from having been awake since ten last night, and the adrenaline of being rushed down the hall to the operating room and the C-section. I was passive for Evelyn's birth as the physicians did the cutting, the pulling, and the sewing of the wound. Yet, I felt as if I had climbed Mt. Kilimanjaro.

The next day, I insisted on walking myself down the two long hallways to see my daughter. "Getting up and walking will help you heal faster," the nurse who offered to push me had said. But she worried about the length I'd have to go to get to the NICU. She asked me to at least walk while pushing a wheelchair so that I'd have some stability, and also so I could sit if I needed to. She allowed Jason to be my companion. My steps were tepid and small, but each one was a pace closer to where I really wanted to be.

My sutures felt like they were tearing open. Standing straight up was impossible. I was still attached to my IV and a catheter, all of which were hooked up to the IV pole Jason pushed down the hall. I couldn't help but wonder why the maternity ward was so far away from the NICU. Didn't they know that mothers need to see their babies? Then, later that day when one of my nurses asked me why my baby wasn't in the room with me, I realized that most babies *are* close to their mothers. Most mothers can see their babies at any time.

When I reached Evelyn's isolette, I sat down in the wheelchair. The nurse handed me a pillow telling me to push it against my stomach. It felt like it was the only thing holding my body together. Evelyn lay there, quiet. Sleeping. Eyes closed. I reached up to the hole in the side of the isolette. Barely reaching her, I touched her tiny hand.

"Can I hold her?" I asked the nurse.

She agreed to bring Evelyn out, but only once the respiratory therapist arrived to help with the CPAP mask. I wrapped my hospital gown around me, trying to cover my back side before sitting back down. My black framed glasses sat on my nose. My hair hadn't been brushed or washed in days.

The respiratory therapist was a young man, with tattooed arms and a gentle smile. He seemed more than happy to reunite a mother with her baby, even if that meant he had to handle something so fragile that it took two of them, him and the nurse, to bring Evelyn out.

When I was settled with the pillow across my lap, the nurse opened the lid of the isolette. She took hold of the cords that ran from the wall to Evelyn's body: several taped to her chest, one that went into her mouth and down her throat, and one attached to a monitor wrapped around her foot. The respiratory therapist held the mask on Evelyn's face, and carefully draped the hose that came off of it onto the floor between us.

"Here she is," he said as he laid her onto the pillow in my lap.

Evelyn's head rested on the inside of my left elbow. Her legs barely reached my right arm.

"Hi, baby," I said. "I'm here now."

"She's been doing great," the respiratory therapist said. "We had to intubate her yesterday for a brief time to get the steroids into her lungs to help make them stronger. But she didn't need that very long."

He smiled down at me, or maybe it was aimed at Evelyn.

"She's a strong one. In fact, she likely won't need the CPAP much longer. Tomorrow her oxygen levels might be stable enough to go down to a nasal cannula."

I didn't know what that meant, but it sounded good. Jason stood over my other side looking down at our daughter.

"Do you want to take our picture?" I asked Jason.

He pulled his phone out of his pocket.

"Do you want a picture with the mask off?" the respiratory therapist asked.

"Can we do that?" I said.

"Sure. For a few moments that would be fine."

He gently peeled the mask back, leaving the elastic band around Evelyn's head. It was the first time I saw up close her eyes, her nose, her mouth, her dainty chin.

"There you are," I said. "Smile for Daddy." Jason took the picture before the respiratory therapist put the mask back on.

"Okay, we should probably put her back in the isolette," the nurse said. I had forgotten she had been patiently waiting on the side, holding the tubes so they wouldn't pull out.

"Of course," I said.

I didn't want to let Evelyn go. I wanted to watch her face, her chest rising and falling with breath, her skin pink with life. But I knew she needed to rest. And so did I.

JOURNEY

We had only been in the NICU for a day or two. Our side of the room was spacious enough for four chairs—the number of visitors allowed at our daughter's bedside at one time. Her monitors were calm. Her heartbeat was steady. Her oxygen level remained above ninety percent, what the NICU nurses said it should be. There was nothing to do but sit.

At times, pockets of the NICU became loud, either with monitor alarms sounding, or the bigger babies crying, or the rustle of family coming through to see the tiny babies. This day, Evelyn's roommate, Journey, had visitors.

"Hi, Mom!" I heard Journey's dad say. He had a strange affectation I'd noticed over the last several days, that the more the situation seemed dire, the more chipper his voice became. It must have been a defense of some kind. "Come on in here."

"How is she? Is she going to be okay?" his mother responded.

I motioned to Jason, tapping him on his arm. Mouthing to him was tough as the curtain didn't stop sound waves.

I pointed.

"No, Mom," the man said almost jovially. "She's not going to be okay." He was trying to not make his mother feel bad for asking. Or he knew his wife was listening, as she always sat quietly by the baby's bedside. But somehow, I suspected it was more than pleasing the others in the room.

"She has something called Trisomy 18, Mom," he said.

"Oh? What's that mean?" she asked.

...

I was told during two separate pregnancies that my baby likely had Trisomy 18, a chromosomal abnormality that literally means there are three of the number 18 chromosomes when there should be two. It causes multiple birth defects and severe cognitive delays. It is reported that ninety percent of babies born with Trisomy 18 die within the first year of life (if they aren't stillborn). It is rare: one out of six thousand births. When we had a chromosomally healthy baby, we ended up rooming with a child who really did have it.

...

I wanted to reach through the curtain and hug the man. I wanted to launch into the full explanation of what I had learned on the Internet about Trisomy 18. I wanted to tell his mother that the baby has a chromosomal problem, that she likely wouldn't survive more than a year (if she even made it out of the NICU), that she would require medical care until her death, that she would never learn to walk, talk, or have the giggle fits babies have. I wanted to tell the grandmother to do as her son was doing. I wanted to tell her to love Journey anyway.

As I listened, I watched Evelyn. She was peaceful. She slept always, hadn't even opened her eyes once. But being two months early, we had to be patient.

...

The night after Evelyn was born, the orthopedic doctor and his nurse came and did an evaluation. Jason and I sat near the curtain. I had learned since her birth the night before that it was best for me to step aside. Let the experts do what they needed to do. What Evelyn needed them to do.

What I didn't know how to do.

At one point, his nurse came over to me. I don't know if she knew I was frightened, or confused, or both. She likely didn't know that we were expecting the joint contractures, but she must have sensed that amongst the chatter at Evelyn's bedside, and our hushed side of the room, she needed to say something.

"She's going to be just fine," the nurse said.

It was the first time, since her birth, a medical professional spoke with optimism.

"Really?" I said.

"We've seen this before. She will just need to be stretched out. Her wrists and knees. But physical therapy can help with that." The nurse patted my knee and smiled.

I thought about the little baby, Journey, across the room. I wondered how, for the first time, we got better news than someone else. Our baby was going to live. Our baby was going to get off of oxygen, out of the isolette, straighten out her wrists and knees and clubfeet. She was going to be *just fine*.

Journey's family would likely never take their daughter home. They would have to leave her behind, her lifeless body, one so tiny and fragile that it just couldn't handle the strain of maintaining a breath or a heartbeat. I saw every day how her mother and father were watching their child slowly die. I imagined them walking out of the hospital empty-handed, just as Jason and I had done four years earlier. I imagined the hopelessness they might feel, just as I had. I also remembered how much love I had felt for Sophia. How the time I spent with her was unexpectedly filled with joy and wonderment.

It wasn't until she stopped breathing that the sorrow came in. I hoped they also felt immense love and admiration for a human so small.

As I watched the orthopedic doctor measure Evelyn's feet, I wished that her family, too, would someday be told that everything would be *just fine*.

ALARMS

The first time Evelyn's oxygen monitor sounded, I jumped in my chair. Jason had been next to mine, checking his phone between chatting with me. At times, he pulled out his tablet and worked through some math that would be part of his post-graduate work.

"Ummm," I said. I searched the room for the origin of the tone. It had never been this loud.

"Yeah," Jason responded. "Should we get someone?"

The sound pierced the air. Surely, it also penetrated the curtains that surrounded each baby.

"Do you think a nurse is going to come?" I asked. I surveyed our half of the room. I pushed aside the curtain that faced the hall and peered out. "Where is someone?" I asked Jason.

Jason rose. His eyes paced.

"I'll be right there!" A nurse poked her head through the curtain. She was on Journey's side. She seemed less panicked than I felt. I wanted that to make me feel better.

When she came over, she skillfully pushed at the buttons. The searing scream stopped. Evelyn was still sleeping.

"There!" she said. She turned. "Was that your first event?"

"Yeah, I think so," I said. Jason had sat back down. We held hands.

"Yeah, this happens all the time around here. Sometimes babies born this small forget to breathe. They stop, their oxygen level drops, and the monitor goes off. Most times, they remember to breathe again on their own and everything is fine."

I thought again to Journey. To how our baby just "forgot to breathe." How, for Journey, it wasn't a matter of just *remembering*: to unclench her fists, to make her heart work right, to correct her erroneous chromosomes.

"All set! Let me know if y'all need anything else!" the nurse said. Her teeth gleamed through her smile.

I wanted to usurp some of her optimism. I wanted to be chipper and nonchalant about these "events."

But all I could do was remember to breathe.

MOVING BABY

About two weeks into Evelyn's stay in the NICU, Jason and I went to the side of the room where Evelyn's isolette was. This morning, unlike the previous fourteen days, Evelyn's bed was gone.

"Oh my god, where's our baby?" I asked Jason.

My eyes darted around the room. I took in the empty floor space, the tiles that were once hidden by her isolette.

"I don't know," he said. "The nurses mentioned that this could happen. That she would have to move up to the NIC2 to make room for new, sicker babies."

I remembered the nurse saying this, how she couldn't tell us specifically when this big move would happen, or where the NIC2 was, or what moving to NIC2 meant for our daughter. All I took away from her was that it would *happen soon*. And to *not worry* when we come in and our child is missing.

Learning not to worry had become a pastime I never wanted to have. It escalated the anxiety I carried with me from childhood. From the discovery that I had Generalized Anxiety Disorder. The recurrence of the ever-present *what if* questions: What if Evelyn's limbs don't straighten out the way they should? What if she never learns how to breathe on her own without "events" and alarms? What if she never learns to feed from a bottle? What if she doesn't ever pass the temperature test—the one where we, or a nurse, puts the thermometer under her armpit every two hours to see if she's maintaining an acceptable body temperature? It was this very test that

Evelyn needed to pass in order to sleep in an open crib, and eventually come home.

Jason and I stood there. I didn't know what else to do. Nothing in the past two weeks had gone the way we thought. Nothing about this pregnancy had been easy.

The curtain was pulled across the room. Journey and her family on the other side were quiet. I looked at the hoses and switches that hung from the wall. For the first time I saw the outlets for the respirators and the bed temperature regulator and the monitors that knew more about our child than we did.

I wanted to cry but knew I really just had to find my baby. Like Jason reminded me, healthier babies went to NIC2. That meant that Evelyn was healthier. Healthier than Journey in the next bed over, healthier than the baby around the circular hallway that was born at twenty-three weeks gestation and was too small, with skin too pink and fragile, to ever come out of his isolette, whose teenage-looking parents sat with him daily, and crossed our paths in the Ronald McDonald breakroom to get their snack of cheese crackers and Coke. Healthier than the baby who died when a virus went around the NICU, the illness from which Evelyn went unscathed.

Evelyn was ready to move to the NICU side that contained the babies born closer to term, the ones who had a heftier birth weight, less trouble breathing, and perhaps just needed a stay of a few days. She was ready to be with the chunky baby who cried all day in his bouncer because he was born with blood sugar regulation issues and probably didn't feel well, and with the new roommate baby who had a deformity with his penis—a detail of his life I didn't need to know but couldn't help but overhear.

Evelyn was ready to take the next step toward going home. For this I knew I should be overjoyed.

But I realized I wasn't ready.

I wasn't ready to let go of the certainty we had finally found in knowing where her isolette would be, the familiarity with the walk down the hallway and the whiteboard that hung just outside her room. I wasn't ready to part with the revolving set of nurses on this side of the NICU—Jeannette, Anne—that I had become fond of. I wasn't ready to let go of the two oversized green recliner chairs that Jason and I wrangled from other parts of the NICU every morning as there was always a shortage. I wasn't ready to never see the view outside of our window again, the one that showed us the top of the next part of the hospital, part of the parking lot, and occasionally a bird that perched on the sill. I wasn't ready to never get a peek at baby Journey across the room. I wasn't ready to face a new walk down the hall, new turns, a new room, new baby roommates, new nurses, new chairs, new views outside of the walls that held my family so tight day after day.

I wasn't ready for Evelyn to move up, move on, and move out of the NICU.

NIC2

Evelyn had to be able to regulate her body temperature before we could leave NIC2. On this side of the NICU, unlike in NIC1 where we started, the machines were quieter, but the babies were louder. They were bigger, more able to cry and wail when they were hungry.

Evelyn's roommates on this side rotated quickly. I supposed that was a good thing: the quicker they got healthy, the sooner they went home. That meant we were also one step closer to going home.

Jim was one of Jason's favorite baby roommates. Jim's mother had other children at home. She worked full-time. She didn't have the summers off teaching like Jason did, or family leave from her job like I did. She didn't have the free time to sit at her baby's bedside every day. As the hours went by, we often looked over at Jim. Always calm, never crying. Once, a napkin that the nurses used as bibs fell onto Jim's face. Jason pointed it out to me and softly walked over there. I giggled. I heard Jason say, "Hey buddy, let me get that for you." He slipped the napkin off.

We weren't at the hospital the day Jim was discharged from NIC2. His mother, a woman we chatted with during the evenings, left us a card with her phone number: *My family has been through the NICU before with my other child. Everything will be okay. Call me if you ever want to talk.*

Jim was replaced with Rhianna, a chunky girl who was always tightly swaddled. For days, we still talked about Jim.

"Jim was my favorite little buddy," Jason said.

LAURA GADDIS

I knew how he felt, watching the babies come and go. Hoping for the best for those we'll never see again. One day, it would be us leaving the others behind.

GOING HOME

Before we could leave the NIC2, Evelyn had to make it through the night without her body temperature dropping. We had tried twice before to open her isolette, and both times her body cooled too much. The third time, it maintained its temperature.

We were then moved to a final room, this time what we called our "private suite." It was a single room with an open-air crib instead of an isolette. We were able to dress Evelyn in the small monkey onesie that we had been gifted by some family who frantically went out to find us preemie clothing before we left that day.

She had passed a series of tests before we made it to this room. They were required before we could go home. First, the eye doctor came around and did his exam. An older nurse had been with us that day. It seemed she had witnessed this many times before.

"It's an exam to make sure the baby's eyes are developed enough. It could detect blindness due to prematurity. But be ready for it," she warned. "It looks worse than it is."

When the ophthalmologist came, he barely greeted us. The nurse laid Evelyn on a blanket-covered cart. He took out his tools and set them down next to Evelyn.

"Hold her please," he said to the nurse.

He picked up one of the instruments, propped open Evelyn's eyelids with his fingers, and dug the metal tool around her eyeball. It was meant to open her eye as wide as possible while he used his scope to look deep within, but it looked like a torture device used in war.

Evelyn wailed. In five weeks, she had barely cried. Not when they took blood from her arms, not when they reinserted her feeding tube through her nose, not when they had to put casts on her tiny legs to fix her club feet.

I looked away.

"Everything looks good," the ophthalmologist said. "In fact, her eyes are nearly as developed as a full-term baby's."

He pulled the instrument from Evelyn's eye. He put away his tools and snapped off his exam gloves.

The nurse grabbed Evelyn, wrapped her back up in the blanket she had ready, and handed her to me. Evelyn laid on my chest. I rubbed her back.

"Shhhh, it's okay, baby. You're all done. It's all done," I said as I wet the top of her head with my tears.

Next, she had to pass the car seat test. This one involved no instruments, except for her car seat. She had to be able to maintain her oxygen level for four hours while sitting, strapped in. Jason and I left for the evening when her nurse did the test. While Evelyn was snoozing, Jason and I found dinner at a nearby restaurant. If she hadn't passed, we'd have had to wait several more days until she was tested again.

The next morning, we were told the good news. In addition to the car seat test, she also passed the hearing exam. I asked little about what that entailed as I didn't think my heart could bear much more. Both were much less challenging than the eye exam. Yet, I was glad I didn't have to sit through another stressful moment.

When we were finally ready to leave the NIC2, the nurse helped us pile up the few pieces of clothes we accumulated for Evelyn, her boppy pillow, and the folder of paperwork that instructed us on how to make follow-up appointments, how to feed her, and how to take care of this baby in the outside world. Then, she put Evelyn, in her car seat, on top of the wheeled cart.

This is how we are going to take her out of here? I thought. *Five weeks of trying to keep her so safe, and she exits on top of a metal cart?*

The cart squealed as we rolled to the elevator. The nurse kept one hand on the handle, one on Evelyn. Part of me wanted to have a celebratory parade as we left the hospital. Another part of me wanted to sneak out quietly before we could make anyone else feel bad. I thought back to the day that Evelyn's roommate, Jim, was discharged. I had been happy for him, and sad for us.

At the elevator, I heard a voice from behind me.

"Are you guys outta here?" said a young mom. She had been the mother of the micro-preemie in NIC1, the 23-weeker. The last time I saw her and her boyfriend, before Evelyn moved to NIC2, they still couldn't take their baby out of the isolette. He was too small, too fragile. They likely wouldn't be leaving anytime soon.

"Yep. And good luck to you guys. I really do hope all goes well with your little one."

"Thank you," she said. "I'm so glad for you guys."

I knew she meant it, even when she sounded sad.

PUMPING

The chair was still in the corner of my office the day I returned to work. Its broad wooden armrests allowed me to balance the milk collection bottles, the valves and membranes, the breast shields and flanges. The cooler bag that held it all together sat on the floor.

Its proximity to the wall outlet made this an ideal place to pump. Ideal in that I had a private room that locked. Ideal in that I could strap on my pumping bra and fit the flanges into the holes without someone walking in on me (probably). Ideal in that it wasn't the bathroom stall, janitorial closet, or the front seat of my car. My sister had to use the office shower stall at her work to pump when her daughter was born five years earlier.

The whirring of the motor was loud. It sounded like a grinding gear, slowly eating away at a piece of chewy bark my lawn mower found in the grass. At times I thought the circular grinding would stop, give out, like a life lost before it could reach its potential.

...

Step 1: Start on low suction. Prime the milk ducts.

Step 2: Slowly increase the suction. Grinding loudens.

Step 3: Wait twenty minutes while the milk is suctioned out of your body, or until you fill both five-ounce bottles (whichever comes first).

Step 4: Don't skimp out on step 3 because the doctor told you your premature baby needs the antibodies to prevent contracting RSV, a life-threatening respiratory illness.

Step 5: Try to score patients' evaluations while the machine grinds the magical fluid from your body. Try to cope with the falling papers and books that fill your lap.

Step 6: Unscrew bottles from tubing, twist on tops (warning: failure to do this may result in loss of magical fluid that only *you* can provide your premature, newborn child), unhook tubes from machine, take flanges off breasts, unhook pumping bra, put on regular bra, pull up/down/fix nursing shirt, stand up and straighten out.

Step 7: Nonchalantly take cooler bag with magical fluid and dirty parts to the fridge, hide milk bottles behind Karen's or Ellen's Yoplait Greek yogurt, go to employee kitchen sink, wash parts. Quickly.

Step 8: Repeat in two to three hours.

Step 9: Repeat seven days a week. Repeat as the summer sun sets earlier and the leaves start to decompose into the soil. Repeat after you feel like you can't, like you don't want to rip more of the skin on your nipples or watch the red painful streaks of mastitis cross your chest. Repeat on holidays: Evelyn's real due date, Jason's birthday, Halloween, Thanksgiving, Black Friday, Christmas Eve, Christmas Day. Repeat on days when coworkers try to open your office door only to find it locked (thank goodness). Repeat after you return to work full-time. Repeat as Evelyn grows chub on her thighs and cheeks. Repeat when eating breakfast, lunch, and dinner. Repeat right before bed at eleven P.M. and again at six in the morning. Repeat until the freezer is full of frozen milk. Repeat until Jason's hands are dry and cracked from the dish soap he uses to wash all the parts. Repeat until the lotion in the house runs out. Repeat until Evelyn starts eating mashed peas and rice cereal. Repeat until the third round of mastitis that is so bad it keeps you in bed. Repeat until you finish the entire regimen of antibiotics, ones that smell like they were made by a farmer scooping up horse manure and shoving it into small plastic capsules, because the doctor told you to help treat mastitis you need to keep pumping through the infection. Repeat until the stockpile of frozen milk is enough to get to Evelyn's first birthday. Repeat until she has come into her own.

CANDLES

Five years earlier, after we came home from the hospital after our first daughter, Sophia's, birth and death, we met my family at our house, and ate Culver's hamburgers. Our small living room was full. Full of hamburgers, full of pickles, full of French fries, full of soda cups, full of straws, full of coats, full of bodies and full of love. Yet, I was empty.

"How do we leave without her?" I had asked Jason a few hours before. We were standing in our hospital room. It was on the recovery floor filled with new mothers, new fathers, and new babies. Our room had only two of the three.

And then, with a house so at-capacity, I had never felt so incomplete.

The birth of my daughter, the holding of her nine-ounce body, the witnessing of her life for an hour-and-a-half eclipsed the fact that it had been New Year's Eve.

Sarah, my sister, brought with her a bag. It was a gift bag, the kind with paper sides and a handle made of twine. When she reached in it, she brought out four tins.

"I thought we could all light a candle for Sophia tonight," she said.

As if I didn't squeeze out enough of my bodily fluids from earlier that day, my eyes let loose a deluge of stale juice left over in the dried-out rinds of my lids.

I lit our candle later that evening, shortly before Jason dug out a lonely, premixed margarita we had in our freezer from a previous gathering (as the discharge nurse had told us to go home and have a glass of wine for New Year's—*if we wanted to, of course*). As the flame danced, the smooth soy wax liquified around the wick. The light was soft. My tears fell. I watched the simplicity of the fire. The teardrop shape. The orange tip and blue base. I remembered from science class in middle school that flames that burned hotter were colored blue, or purple. I wondered if the blue knew that the wick wouldn't last forever. That the wax would melt, and the scent of lilies would evaporate into the air. I wondered if the blue still felt invincible.

I wondered if the candle would soothe my heartbreak as the aroma soothed my senses. If I had known about rainbow babies then, if I had had the chance to read about success after loss, if my innocence about pregnancies had been lost before now, I could have also wondered if, had the light hit my tears in just the right way, at just the right angle, would it produce a rainbow? To have such hope at such a time of hard grief seemed impossible. Now, I think back and suspect that I would have loved that thought.

...

For the next several years, Sarah sent candles. Even when one was not completely used from the previous year, a new one would shine. We gathered a collection. Tins of pink, silver, green, black swirls. As we had moved several times over the years since Sophia's birth, the tins found themselves in various boxes. The ninth Christmas after Sophia's birth (and death), we put up our tree in Ohio. It would be the final home that Jason and I planned to make. He finally had a tenure-track job, and I returned to school. Evelyn was enrolled in preschool and daycare, had physical therapists, an occupational therapist, an orthopedic doctor, teachers, and friends. She had many friends. Friends that loved her for just how she was; with braces on her legs, a stiff-gaited walk, and a giggle so infectious they couldn't help but fall into a pile on the carpet when her little buddies came over to play.

"We are home, candles," I found myself whispering as I unpacked two, one with a green label and another with a pink one. My sister had texted a few days prior saying she couldn't afford gifts this year. *Let's just get the girls presents, if that's okay with you,* she had said. I had no problem acquiescing to such a request. She was recently single, previously divorced, and had an eight-year-old to raise.

But when her presents came in the mail for Evelyn, amongst them was one pink-and-white box. It was labeled for Jason, for Evelyn, and for me. It was our candle.

CRITERIA I NEED TO MEET TO SELF-DIAGNOSE (PART 3 OF 4)

Criterion 4[23]: The anxiety and worry are accompanied by at least three additional symptoms from a list that includes restlessness, being easily fatigued, difficulty concentrating, irritability, muscle tension, and disturbed sleep.

Jason, Evelyn, and I had just moved to a small townhouse in Oxford, Ohio with three bedrooms, one living room, and an eat-in kitchen. Evelyn was now two. Jason began his job at Miami University while

---

[23] I need naps daily around one pm and I have always tired easily (I worry when I won't be home for hours at a time: beginning of the year school shopping; vacations that include a lot of walking, hiking, waiting in line for rides; going to shows/movies/classes in the middle of the afternoon); I'm especially fatigued when nervous—I yawned in a constant stream whenever I had to play clarinet or piano solos in front of a judge or an audience of parents, or when I had to do a presentation for class, or when I had a doctor's appointment scheduled; when my thoughts were tied to other worries, I often lash out at my husband when I am not *really* mad at him; frequent (daily, really) headaches, tensed facial and neck muscles; clenched thighs and buttocks when in situations where I feel out of control like in the passenger seat of a moving car; insomnia (not able to fall asleep *and* not staying asleep); dreams about terrible things like my sister dying, or me being chased, or me falling, or my daughter disappearing; and, periods of time where I wake up at two A.M. and don't fall back asleep until I quiet the racing thoughts around four A.M. Damn.

I had moved here with no job prospects or even an idea of what I could do. I had left my job as a psychometrist when we left North Carolina behind. It was a relief to quit, a relief to clean up my office of: framed photos of Evelyn, and of Jason and me posing at a restaurant, my few books on psychopathology, and my testing clipboard lined with stats and charts and formulas on how to calculate averages and standard deviations. Eight years of conducting psychological evaluations on children and adults had become tiresome. I carried many heavy stories. Adults in their fifties with early-onset Alzheimer's learning that their rate of disease progression was rapid, and they had maybe a year (or two at best) to continue their world travels. Children with severe autism who lacked verbal skills, social skills, and would likely never be potty-trained. A man who sustained a brain injury from a car accident, unable to control his anger, throwing a pencil across the table at me when he couldn't answer a question. I was tired.

Still, I didn't know what I would do with the next thirty years until I reached retirement age.

That was equally as heavy.

Within the first couple of months in our Ohio home, I began waking up at two A.M. I tossed and turned, trying my right ear on the pillow, then my left. I counted to one hundred. I sang songs to myself. I played soft nature sounds from my phone's meditation app. I often got up and retreated to the couch downstairs. I covered myself up with my large pink blanket, one that Jason had gifted me one Christmas when we still lived in North Carolina. It was my favorite; the softness soothed my skin and the large size covered my body with plenty of extra to wrap around me and tuck.

By four A.M., I fell back asleep. At six, my alarm went off to start another day—a day of getting Evelyn up and dressed for daycare, of prepping for teaching my introduction to psychology course, of slogging through the hours as I made breakfast, lunch, and dinner, of walking the dog, giving Evelyn her evening baths, dressing her in pajamas, putting her to bed, and trying again to sleep another night.

THERAPY

When we first moved to Oxford, I was driving Evelyn to her new daycare, sobbing as we drove down College Ave. The cobblestone section of road masked the sniffles and guttural throat rumbles, until the pavement turned to asphalt.

"Why are you crying, Mommy?" Evelyn asked from the backseat.

"It's nothing, baby. Don't worry about it."

I didn't want my anxiety to burden her. I didn't want her to think about how Jason and I had moved three times in the past five years and that each time was to a new state, a new city, a new home to unpack our lives from the boxes they were reduced to. I didn't want her to think *she* was a burden, her weak muscle tone, her legs that refused to let her walk without a walker. I didn't want her to have to worry about who her new physical therapist would be, how the in-home therapy worked in the state of Ohio and the emails I had sent to someone named "Ann" and another named "Sandy" and yet a third named "Stephanie" just to figure out how to get my daughter services, how we'd have to find a new orthopedic doctor after we had to leave a fantastic one behind in North Carolina, who her new pediatrician would be, who her new teachers would be and if they could handle a child with physical limitations. I didn't want her to feel the stress of living in a small town where we knew only two people (the professor that recommended Jason for the job and his wife) and we were at least five hours from the nearest family member. I didn't want her to know that my anxiety, the kind that takes every moment of the day and bloats it up with angst and worry and hypotheticals, had reached a peak until I couldn't help but cry while driving her to school.

Evelyn was sitting happily in the backseat. The weather was sunny and mild. The traffic was barely there. Yet, I cried. I didn't want her to realize that I cried at my overcrowded thoughts. That I cried when I was home alone after Jason had left to teach for the day. And that I cried in the shower, in the kitchen, and at night as I tried to sleep. I didn't want her to know about the worries that woke me up most nights. It was during this car ride that I decided to find a therapist.

...

Before leaving my house for my first appointment with Jennifer, I had been watching the time tick down to the moment I had to leave. The tears that formed were my body's way of calming down, yet they didn't make me feel better. I couldn't articulate why they came. The salty tracks probably smudged my mascara. Dark lines probably lined my cheeks. Flecks of black makeup residue likely outlined my eyelids. But I couldn't care. I needed to leave. With only ten minutes until my appointment time, I now feared I would be late getting to a place Google Maps said was five minutes away. I had to leave time for stop lights, rogue pedestrians, or suicide squirrels running out in front of my car. I had to leave time for getting stuck behind drivers turning left. I had to leave time to navigate the office building, the two floors and one set of stairs. I had to leave time to breathe once I parked, but before I could get out of the car.

I had to go.
1. Find my wallet and keys.
2. Put them in my purse.

3. Get into my car in the garage.
4. Open the garage.
5. Get into the driver's seat.
6. Put the key in ignition.
7. Start the car.
8. Back out of the garage.
9. Close the garage.
10. Put the car into 'drive'.
11. Press the accelerator.
12. Go to the person who could help.
13. Any more than one step at a time, and I was sure I would lose my breath and pee myself.

...

I almost cancelled the appointment. Not because I didn't want the help, but because the idea of coming to this office—a place I hadn't seen before, in a building I hadn't been in before, meeting a person I had never talked to before, and being seen by the other workers from the Remax realtor's office and the insurance office that shared the space with the counseling office—made me taste the bile that rose from my stomach. If only I weren't afraid of making a phone call or of having to talk to someone I didn't know. Or, it was this anxiety that did me a favor for once.

...

The waiting room fit two chairs and a small table between them. An electric fireplace crackled in the corner. The television above it played meditative music and water ripples. The clipboard was waiting for me on the table. My name was on it, but just the first name because,

HIPAA again, you know. I was the lone person. A button sat on the table inscribed with "click once" and "Jennifer" in black marker. My breathing slowed a bit. It was comforting to know I was expected. It was comforting knowing I made it in unseen by the realtors and insurance agents. I grabbed the clipboard, a pen, and a small peanut butter cup from the candy dish.

...

Please fill out the following:

1. What is your main concern?

~~I worry.~~ (*but who doesn't?*) ~~I worry A LOT.~~ (*what does a lot even mean?*) I have a lot of anxiety about a lot of things and don't know how to control it.

2. What do you hope to gain from therapy?

~~I want to be more calm~~ (*who doesn't want to be more calm? That doesn't seem legit.*) I feel like I am overly out-of-control with my anxiety, and I want to be able to be like everyone else. I want to be able to enjoy things more without worrying about them.

3. Have you ever sought treatment in the past?

❏ Yes

x No

4. Have you ever taken medication for depression or anxiety?

❏ Yes

x No

...

With the form complete, my thoughts returned to the lobby door, to the creaky steps leading back upstairs, to my car sitting outside in the parking lot, awaiting my return. The same Toyota Matrix that took me to all of my prenatal appointments, to the hospital the night my Sophia was born and died, to ultrasounds and blood tests. It was also the car that always returned me home, safely, at the end. I considered ways of getting back to my car without being noticed. I almost left the room before Jennifer came to get me.

The door opened. A golden Labrador's head poked out. His panting reminded me of my pug's.

The dog made me smile.

"Laura?"

"Yes."

"Hi! I'm Jennifer. And this is Milo," she said pointing down to the lab. "Come on back. I'm the second door on the right."

Jennifer appeared to be in her thirties, had long brown hair, was tall and fit. She wore a blouse and skirt, similar to the dress code I followed in all of my past psychology jobs. She did not wear bangle bracelets like Judith, my former therapist, had. I couldn't distract myself within the red lipstick and the smoker's hack that I could with Judith.

I didn't know how to explain to this woman my lifetime of constant worries. Or where they may have come from. *Just try, Laura. Do this for you. And for Evelyn.*

"Tell me about why you are here," Jennifer said as we walked into her office. I chose the chair that sat next to a small side table. The couch seemed too big, too engulfing. It was furthest away from the chair Jennifer sat in. Would she wonder why I chose the couch, so far away, if I sat there? Was the couch meant for couples, or those whose bodies couldn't be comfortably sat in the chair? Was this a test to see how much space I put between her and me, the anxious one and a stranger?

Of course, it's a test, I thought. *It usually is. How far do you sit away from the therapist (when she's a stranger, then after three weeks of sessions, then a year later)? What is your body language—arms crossed over your chest? Guarded behind walls of limbs? Sitting on the edge of your chair or leaning back on the extra pillows?* All were behavioral observations I made notes of while working with my patients. Jennifer, too, would certainly be making those notes about me.

Milo brought his rawhide up to me, dropped it at my feet, an offering of acceptance. His head was soft under my fingertips.

"Hi, buddy," I said. He jumped his front paws on my lap. *It's a good thing my anxiety doesn't include big dogs.*

"Milo, down. Go to your bed," Jennifer said. He sulked away. I wanted to curl up with him on his floor pillow.

I crossed my legs but not my arms. My hands rested on the leather armrests, pretending to be casual under the sweat. When my hand moved away, my palm print remained. Jennifer looked down to take notes on her iPad (likely about my posture, my positioning, my sweat, my shaking leg). I wiped the residual hand away.

"Well..." I had to think for a moment. "I see other people going about their lives, doing things, going places, meeting people, and they seem to do it without much fear. They actually seem to *enjoy* themselves."

Jennifer nodded. She kept writing.

"I feel like I can't do that. I worry all the time about everything. I know it's dumb, and that most of my worries are not true. But I can't stop it. I feel like I'm over *here*," I motioned with my hands to the left. "And everybody else is over *there*." I motioned to the right. "I want to be over there, too."

...

Over the course of sessions every two to three weeks, Jennifer helped me acknowledge that biology was likely behind my anxiety (partly). My mom and I exhibited the same panic, the same demands for control, down to the same worries about entering new restaurants (and making someone else go first). I likely inherited this partially, and also learned it behaviorally, observationally.

...

Albert Bandura, an American psychologist, described observational learning where a child learns behaviors, emotions, and attitudes from the major adult figures in a child's life. In his social learning theory, he goes on to describe four necessities for observational learning to work:

1. **Attention:** *if a child is not paying attention to the adult figure, whether it be because of sleepiness, or attention-sustaining difficulties*

due to disorders such attention deficit hyperactivity disorder, or is otherwise distracted, learning of the behaviors will not occur.

On a trip to visit my sister in Madison, Wisconsin my dad, mom, grandmother and I all rode in a car together. It was raining, the drops pounding harder the further west we drove. Finally, the drops became sheets of rain, blinding us from any more than a few feet in front of the car. Through the water my mom saw the red taillights in front of us.

"Slow down!" she yelled. Her fist pounded the dashboard. "Slow down, slow down!"

"It's fine," my dad said. My father's tempered response seemed a learned reaction to my mother's outbursts.

"You need to slow down!" My mom's voice maintained its loudness, its high tone, its panic.

My grandma took my hand across the middle-back seat. When I leaned over, I could see the heavy rain, the lights, the dark outline of the car appearing in front of us. I could see just how close we were to the car, but also saw that my dad did, indeed, stop in time.

My mom's tone rattled me. I didn't notice the car in front until she yelled. I didn't fear my dad's reaction to the drenching rain until she pounded the dashboard. I didn't know to be fearful until she showed me how. My heart rate increased, my breathing ragged, and I knew in that instant how she felt, why she screamed when she didn't need to, when she could have trusted my dad to be the safe driver that he had always been.

2. Retention: *the observer must remember the witnessed event to have a greater chance of imitating it.*

Over twenty years later, my muscles still tense in the car when it rains. The first droplets on the windshield make the familiar tensing in my thighs begin, and when the droplets morph into a shower into a downpour into a drenching, my buttocks lock together, and my hand grip causes sore knuckles.

Over twenty years later, I still remember the car ride to Madison. The rain, the yelling, the hand pounding the front of the car, the red lights, the way my grandma held my hand.

3. Reproduction: *the observer of the behavior must be able to exhibit, or reproduce, the same behavior. The observer must be physically and mentally able to copy the actions.*

Shortly after moving to Baltimore, Maryland with Jason, we decided to drive to visit my parents in Wisconsin. We left after Jason was done teaching for the day. The western half of Maryland is rugged where the Bear Pond and Allegheny Mountains meet just northwest of Hagerstown, Maryland. It was early spring. The darkness came early in the evening, especially by the time we drove the three hours to the beginning of the mountain roads. The air was thin and cold near the top of each drive upward, the warm spring air condensing into fog on the road as the altitude rose.

"Be careful!" I said.

"I am being careful, babe," said Jason.

"I know, but just be careful… please."

The car wound past trees that lined the sides. Beyond our headlights, I could see nothing. No pavement. No yellow lines. Not a car, a deer, a rabbit, or a fallen rock.

"Oh my god, we can't see anything. Please be careful!" My hand gripped the door handle. My buttocks clenched, as if holding my muscles taut could slow the car.

"I'm doing the best I can, babe. Please stop yelling." Jason's voice was tense but would have likely been terser if he hadn't been concentrating so hard on the road.

I breathed in and out, I averted my eyes to my legs where they couldn't see the tiny white droplets that formed the nearly opaque cloud that surrounded us.

"It's getting better," Jason said.

"Are we going down the mountain now?" My eyes squeezed shut.

"Yep. I can definitely see better." He grabbed my hand and held it over the console. My buttocks relaxed. I could finally let go. Until we went up again, and back down.

That night we stayed at a La Quinta in Xenia, Ohio. I had never been so grateful to be on the flat plains of middle Ohio, nearing the flatter lands of Indiana and Illinois.

3. Motivation: *perhaps the most important element to observational learning, the observer has to witness a benefit, or believe in a benefit, to copying a behavior. Negative consequences can also work to lessen a behavior. If an observer sees the adult being punished for a behavior, it is less likely to be copied.*

I'm not sure I ever figured out what benefits my mom got from hitting the dashboard or yelling "stop!" repeatedly at the driver. Perhaps the benefits were more internal; her pleas calmed her brain, increased the likely lowered serotonin levels (or that was what she hoped it would do).

There was never a visible downside. My dad remained calm. We didn't hit the car in front of us. My mom was able to calm down once we drove out from under the other side of the raincloud. While it's not clear that her behaviors did anything to resolve the situation, or that she believed they did, that connection could be made, subconsciously or not. My brain may have made the same connections and retained those behaviors for the later date in the mountains.

...

To acknowledge the etiology of my anxiety was freeing. There was likely a genetic component, a strong link to the predisposition for my mind to not create enough serotonin, a neurotransmitter that regulates mood and depression, levels of anxiety, sleep habits, appetite, memory, irritability. It is produced in both the brain and the intestines, but the majority (95%) comes from the gut. Some people, people like my mom and me, may just produce less serotonin than others. Perhaps it is due to having fewer serotonin receptors. Or not. It is not well understood, but it does seem to have a strong biological factor. If my mom did have a serotonin deficit, and so did I, I didn't blame her. Just as I didn't blame my dad's Norwegian roots for my blue eyes, blond hair, and skin so fair that it burns within ten minutes of being in the summertime sun, and blisters in thirty.

Perhaps I passed it to Evelyn. Maybe she, too, will panic in the car when she notices a second before the driver that the car in front of her puts on the brakes and she, too, will say "watch out!" and put a hand to the dashboard. Or she will wake at two A.M., brain racing through what she needs to do tomorrow—fill out school forms for her child, call the doctor to make a well-visit appointment for herself and her daughter, take the dog to the vet for his Bordetella vaccine before our next vacation, finish the laundry that had piled up in the hamper, read half a novel for her graduate class that she needs to have done by the end of the week, find a job in a new town, or wonder if she locked the front door after coming in from her evening walk.

Once I recognized this, gained the insight that my body's chemicals may be off and affected how I had lived for most of my life, I allowed Jennifer to help.

...

My parents had come to visit us in Ohio. We sat around the small pine dining table in the eat-in kitchen of our first rented home in Oxford. It was big enough to seat four people. Five of us crowded around.

"I saw the last piece you wrote on your blog talked about anxiety," my mom said. I thought, *she'll see our connection. She'll see my behavior in her. Maybe I will finally have someone who understands what it's like to be me.*

"Yeah, it's something I've been dealing with since I was a kid. I don't know if you remember how anxious I would get about things."

"Maybe a little," my mom said.

"I really didn't notice," said my dad.

I was surprised and a little disappointed that they didn't seem to recognize this part of me, a core trait that has been with me for as long as I could remember. But then I had to remind myself that they weren't *me*. They didn't live my life, but, instead, were observers. Only *I* could see my anxiety for what it truly was. And only I could make a change.

"Well, I still struggle with it, so I thought I'd try and get some help." I said. I now knew what I had to do to become a better version of myself.

...

On subsequent visits to my parents, I watched my mom pour her orange juice into a cup that held six ounces. She always drank it with one rectangular ice cube that filled the glass nearly to the top.

"If I take one pill, then how many will be left?" she asked Evelyn.

"One, two, three, four…" Evelyn said. "Six!"

"That's right! I had seven, and take one away, and have six."

Evelyn watched my mom swallow the pill. She observed the way Nana put it on her tongue on a place to the side (because too much in the middle made her gag, she once told me). The way she took a small sip of her juice, held it in her mouth for two or three seconds. The way she held her fist up to her mouth before the gulping noise happened. The way she looked away for a moment while she prepped for the next pill.

"Now what?" Evelyn asked.

"Now I take this one."

"What about this one here?" Evelyn asked pointing to a large white tablet.

"That one I save for last. It's the hardest to take."

One by one, my mom took a pill, and they counted down.

"Well, I ran out of juice for this last one," my mom said.

"But you need to take it!" said Evelyn.

"I don't have anything to take it with," my mom said.

"You could get a little more juice," I said. Sitting at the far end of the counter, I had stayed out of their conversation up until now. I had confessed to Jennifer that my reactions to my mom sometimes turned into a power struggle. I wanted to be right, to change her behaviors, to make her see things my way. This rigidity was mine to own. And I was ready to change it. Jennifer advised when I noticed those moments to pause and step away.

Here I was, in a moment Jennifer and I had talked about—a moment with a solution so simple, yet my mom chose to do something else. It is this kind of moment that made me vocally question my mom when I was younger, the kind of moment that I used to bait her into an argument that blew up into something far bigger than it ever should have been.

"I only drink one glass with my breakfast. I'll just save this one for my breakfast tomorrow," she said.

I smiled.

I nodded.

I thought of saying *what's wrong with getting just a little more juice?*

I thought of saying *it seems ridiculous to let one pill go until tomorrow.*

I thought of saying *are you sure you'll have enough juice tomorrow to take it after all of tomorrow's pills?*

I said, "Okay."

...

I wanted Evelyn to see me letting go of what didn't need to be, to see me making my own choices, making the choice not to press the fact that getting a bit more juice would have been more logical with little downside. I wanted Evelyn to see my flexibility, my ability to turn my attention to something I could control (like the crossword puzzle I was filling in). I wanted Evelyn to know that she may not be able to control others, and that others will always have influences on her, but she has power. Power in herself, in her own actions, in her own choices of when to fight, when to say something, when to worry, when to pound the dashboard, and when none of that is necessary. I wanted Evelyn to be free from the shackles that have kept me tied to my fears, to my defensiveness, even if she had to learn that from watching me find my own way.

THE YELLOW BRACES

Five years after losing my first baby, I found myself sitting on my couch next to my daughter putting on her ankle-foot orthotics (AFOs) while she watched Daniel Tiger's Neighborhood. The braces were not the new ones she was supposed to be wearing, but they still worked to keep her ankles from rolling and the edges of her feet becoming the soles they weren't meant to be. I struggled to pull apart the plastic to make the opening in the front of each boot-like apparatus expand beyond the width of her foot.

"Ow!" Evelyn said. I had barely gotten her foot inside, but I could feel the scraping of the plastic edge along her socked heel.

"I'm sorry, baby," I said.

What I really wanted to say was:

I hate these damn things!
I wish you didn't have to wear them!
I never want to have to put these stupid braces on your feet again.
I'm doing the best that I can!
Work with me!
I'm sorry you have to wear these.
We'll be doing this FOREVER!
We HAVE been doing this forever!
Maybe, just maybe, someday, you won't have to wear them.

Oh god, I hope there is a day you don't have to wear them. (Is that a prayer?)

I pulled the yellow Velcro (all three bands) over the front of her braces to keep them in place. The "Pringles," as they are called because of their shape, fit snugly on top of her ankle joint to keep her skin from becoming red and irritated. When she was a baby and wore different braces—the Ponseti shoes—twenty-three-hours a day, we didn't have the Pringles. The leather straps on those rubbed her skin into delicate flaps of useless protection. Her ankles had become raw. The doctor told us that over time, these wounds would become scars. The redness would last forever. I had called the orthotics place later that day and got Pringles for those braces. Her skin slowly grew back together. The red blotches returned to peach.

The yellow straps of her AFOs accompanied the Tweety Birds she chose for the plastic decoration. The foam on the inside was yellow. When we did the fitting at her physical therapist's office for these, she was shown all the color and pattern options.

"Yellow, yellow, yellow," Evelyn had said.

I was not surprised my child chose the brightest color possible. Three times.

But now, the color couldn't make me less bitter about what we had to do every day. The struggle to put on her braces, even though she cooperated most of the time. The struggle to find tennis shoes, or any shoes, that would fit over them. The struggle to not clip her foot between the plastic edges every damn time. The struggle in watching her walk with a steadier gait at the expense of not being able to jump, walk on her tiptoes, or run properly as the plastic held her ankles in a secure L-shape. The struggle to convince her sometimes to put her shoes back on after a nap because she wanted to be barefoot like her friends. Like her mommy who walked around the house sans shoes. The struggle to convince myself that this is the best for my child when I see others run and play so free.

Now her braces were on.

I took the left Paw Patrol tennis shoe and stretched it out. I pulled the tongue out. I pulled the sides apart. I straightened the heel of the opening as it always folded in on itself as we pulled it over her braced foot. I slid her toes in first, making sure they were as far to the front of the shoe as possible. I pulled at the tongue, keeping it sticking out the top as if it were a child's face mocking my efforts. I wiggled her foot with one hand while trying to be gentle, to not squeeze her ankle too hard with the other. I slid the heel a bit over the end of the plastic, stopped, wiggled her foot, slid the shoe, stopped, wiggled her shoe until her heel hit the bottom. I pushed the tongue back down to clear the way for the Velcro strap. I pulled it tight.

One shoe was on. One more to go. Repeat after nap later in the afternoon. Repeat tomorrow morning. And the next…and the next…

"Thanks, Mommy," Evelyn said as she swung her legs back to the edge of the couch. Her eyes had never left Daniel Tiger practice riding his bike.

Evelyn rode her tricycle every day. She began pedaling for longer stretches, her thigh muscles bulking up in strength to make up for the low tone she was born with. Once at the top of the hill, at the end of the block, at the stop sign she has come to know as the place to turn around, she whizzed her trike down the middle of the empty street saying, "catch me, Mama!"

The Paw Patrol shoes, the yellow-yellow-yellow plastic, the Pringles all make that possible.

As I got up from the couch, I left her with Daniel Tiger. I kissed her forehead. "Of course, baby."

I walked back to the kitchen. I found my coffee cup. Daniel's voice softened in the background. The last bit of coffee was lukewarm. The almond milk that had been carefully mixed with the coffee was now separating into a settling swirl toward the bottom of the mug. On top, I could only see the remnants of white. They clung to the surface. They struggled to stay where I put them, to float when they felt the urge to drown. I took my spoon and swirled the liquid, making the dark brown light again.

ERASURE

The week before we left on a trip to visit my parents, Evelyn asked, "How many days until we leave to see Nana and Papa?"

She was five years old and was beginning to understand that my parents, her Nana and Papa, lived in Wisconsin, far from our Ohio home.

"It's like…" I counted on my fingers, partly for me, partly for her to understand and hopefully not ask this question repeatedly for the next week. "…. six days."

"Yay!" Evelyn said.

"And remember, Evelyn," I said, "It's a long ride to Nana and Papa's house."

"How long? Like to Aldi?"

"No, baby," I laughed. "That's only like twenty-five minutes away. Nana and Papa are like five or six hours away."

"Why are you laughing?" Evelyn asked.

"Nothing, sweetie. I wish Nana and Papa lived like Aldi away."

"Me too."

Two years after Evelyn's birth in Winston-Salem, North Carolina, Jason had finally reached the point in his mathematics career (after graduate school, a year in San Diego as a visiting assistant professor, and a three-year stint at Wake Forest University in a post-doc) that he was hirable for a tenure-track mathematics professor job. When he first told me about Miami University, located in a small town in southwest Ohio, I said, "I don't want to go there!" But this move (hopefully the last one) got Jason the best thing to a dream job, it got Evelyn close to the physical therapists, occupational therapists, and orthopedic doctors at Cincinnati Children's Hospital, and it got me seven hours closer to my family. We were finding our way home.

...

The trip to my parents' house stretched out over six hours, as we stopped twice to use the restroom, and once more to eat lunch at Culver's. A butter burger and custard were a sure sign we were approaching Milwaukee. I remembered the warm summer Wisconsin evenings, the kind that only lingered around during July and August (and June and September if we were lucky) when my mom, dad, sister, and I would venture out to Kopps Custard stand. Kopps was the precursor to the Culver's chain. The only three locations were in the Milwaukee area (Greenfield, Brookfield, Glendale). The Greenfield location was the closest to our house, and catered to the warmer Wisconsin days with its outside seating on cement benches in a courtyard with decorative flower beds, trees, and a wall at the far end that had a stream of water falling over the edge and into the side pool below. The burgers were as large as the bottom of a coffeepot, the custard (*not* ice cream according to any Midwesterner) was thick, smooth, and tasted as if they had frozen a carton of pure heavy cream. We had taken Evelyn to Kopps once on a previous trip. There was photographic evidence of her chocolate-ringed mouth as she sat on a bench in the Kopps' courtyard near the waterfall.

At my parents' house, I helped Evelyn climb down from her car seat.

"We're here! We're here!" she said.

"Yes, sweetie, but calm down. I don't want you to fall."

She couldn't yet run, her legs moved stiffly, only her left knee bending slightly with each step while her right knee remained locked. It was the same leg, though, that kicked the back of my seat repeatedly during the last hour of the ride as she asked *are we getting closer?*

"Remember to try bending your knees a little when you walk!" I said. "It'll help you go faster."

"And watch out for the bump in the sidewalk!"

"I know, Mama!" Evelyn had taken off around the side of the garage. Her arms swung as if she were downhill skiing, yet instead of wielding poles, their empty motions helped keep her balanced. Her left arm moved freely. Her right arm swung a smaller arc, most of the movement coming from her elbow. She lifted her shoulder with each movement, tilting her body so that her arm could go higher, faster, farther.

The garage was dark except for one dim bulb that came on when it sensed motion.

"Watch your step in here, Ev. It's a little dark."

"I'm okay!"

"Be careful with the step inside. You can use the handle that Papa put on the wall for Oma to use."

"I don't need that!"

"Then give me your hand." I took it before she could respond. She swung her right leg outward, doing what her physical therapist called *circumventing* to get her leg up on the step.

"It's a way to compensate for her inability to lift from her hip flexor and pull up at her knee," Ms. Nicole had told us.

Evelyn pushed hard on her right leg, the sole of her foot now planted solidly on the ground, said *"uuuhhh,"* and pulled her left leg up to match.

MOSAIC

Once up the two steps, she returned to her wild gait. Her knees did not yield to my suggestion of bending.

...

This was the second house of my childhood—one my engineer father had planned at the drawing table at the old house and my artist mother helped to conceive. The drawing table sat in the basement, in the space between the well-lit laundry room and the darkened end used for storage. This table had been a fixture in my childhood. It was similar to one that my father used when he hand-drew large mining machinery for his company, Bucyrus-Erie. It was the table my mom used when she worked on her fine art. She painted, often with watercolor, here. Once, she made a picture of a blue and red swirl with her airbrush (in some medium I didn't know) and then erased where a penguin should be. The white became the picture. I often stared at that penguin, fascinated by the idea of creating something by taking something away.

...

Some poets create *erasure* or *blackout* poetry. The artist uses this technique to obscure large portions of text to create an entirely different text. It is a form of *found* poetry; finding something in something else; finding new meaning in an old one. When I lost my first baby, I *found* new emotions: profound grief, traumatic fears of more loss, deep sadness. I also *found* myself writing and creating and expressing myself in new ways.

The erasure penguin had seemed beautiful to me all those years ago. Now, I understood why.

...

"Nana! Papa! Eeeeee!"

"Hi, sweetie!" My mom and dad were sitting on their stools at the kitchen counter.

"Hi, Evelyn!" she said again, this time getting up from her stool. My mother had always chosen the stool at the end of the peninsula counter so she could get up easily to reach things from the kitchen. My dad always sat next to her. Then came me. Then my sister. Always.

My mom's knees, ankles, feet, and hips were relatively unscathed from her rheumatoid arthritis. I don't remember a time that my mother's pills (the yellow ones, the translucent ones, the blue ones, and the small pile of white ones) weren't lined up near her placemat. The mixture of colors changed every day. Some days there were more pills than others. They kept her rheumatoid arthritis under control. Even with the fingers of her right hand pointed at an angle, the knuckles swollen like marbles under her skin, these pills had kept her from being nearly chair-bound as I remember her once being. There was a time the pain in her hips made walking too difficult. These pills kept her moving.

"Nana!"

My mom stooped down to hug Evelyn. She was the only family member in the older generation, except for Jason's mom (also 'nana') that could still get on the floor, and *would* get on the floor.

"How are you, Evelyn?"

"Good," Evelyn said. Then with her arms still wrapped around her nana, her head resting on my mom's shoulder, she added, "Do you want to play?"

...

When my parents designed their house, they likely didn't imagine they would share it with a grandchild. They likely didn't imagine Evelyn playing with her Legos on the family room floor or swimming in the inflatable zebra kiddie pool in the backyard. When we visited, Evelyn slept in the library—a former bedroom that once belonged to my sister. The sky-blue plush carpet had been replaced with a green and yellow vine-patterned one. Where Sarah's bed once was now stood a small flat-panel TV on a half-circle table. The computer and desk chair approximated where her dresser and desk were. My old room became the guest room. I dubbed it the 'ivy room' as my mom had painted thin ivy leaves along the oval outline of the tray ceiling. My teal carpet, the one I chose as a middle-school child, remained. The dried glue spot, from where I had accidentally tipped over an Elmer's bottle, orange cap not quite turned all the way closed, was gone.

...

Sunday was what my mom called the 'big pill day.' Methotrexate kept her arthritis under control. She had to take five of them twice on Sundays. That was in addition to the fish oil she had read would help sustain her memory, and vitamins to keep her from catching colds, and others I never knew the identity of.

When Jason and I were first married and childless, he replaced Sarah on the last stool at the counter. Now Evelyn often sat in my mom's spot, my mom relenting to the lower, backless stool they bought for times when there would be more than four of us. Times when we might be missing my sister but adding my daughter. Times when the stool assignments were erased and became something new.

"What are these pills, Nana?"

"Those are just different medicines and vitamins I need to take to stay healthy," said my mom.

"Why so many? Can we count them?" Evelyn said. "One, two, three…"

"How many are there?" my mom asked.

"Five!"

"Yes! Very good! Five white ones because today's my big pill day."

My mom had been diagnosed when I was too young to remember. Eventually, the movement she had in her fingers was replaced with a stiffness. Even so, she had always refused to get infusions. She resisted surgery. And she found ways to carry on.

…

Watching my mom and Evelyn count the pills reminded me of grocery shopping as a kid. She always carried a little pocket calculator in her purse. When there was a sale, my mom asked me to calculate what the reduced price would be.

"Multiply the original price by the percent off. Remember to make the percent into a decimal first. Then we'll know how much to subtract to get the sale price," she said.

Another time, we determined which size shampoo bottle was the better deal per ounce.

"Divide the price by the number of ounces in this bottle. What did you get? Oh, good. Remember that number. Now do the same for this bottle. Okay, which is less expensive per ounce?"

We were always figuring out what we could gain by taking something away.

MOSAIC

...

On the Sunday after we arrived at my parents' house, my mom was doing laundry. It used to be on Saturday mornings. But aside from the one-day shift, nothing had changed. Laundry started early, as soon as she was up in the morning. When I was a teenager and would be at the movies with my friends late on a Friday night, sleeping until nine the next morning, she said *please put out your laundry tonight!* so she could start it at eight. If she forgot to tell me, a sticky note with the message would be waiting on the railing to the upstairs. She sorted the clothes into more piles and loads than I ever could get used to doing for myself: whites, lights, darks, jeans. She preferred to hang-dry all of her clothes (except for the whites) and had a special line installed over the back porch. It retracted when not in use, giving the illusion of the laundry never having been there. Even when it was a forty-degree day in Wisconsin, my mother texted me *I got my laundry out today!* I wondered if she still folded her shirts one arm at a time and rolled sock pairs into balls. I assumed she did.

This Sunday she asked Evelyn, "Do you want to help me hang laundry?"

"Yes!" Evelyn said.

"Okay, let's go outside."

When they returned, my mom declared, "Evelyn did a great job handing me the clothespins. She chose the colors and everything."

"I did a good job, Mama!"

"Good, Evelyn. Thanks for helping Nana."

My mom added, "Evelyn said she had never seen a clothespin before, so I had to show her how it worked."

"Yeah…" I said. "I don't really hang my clothes."

A year earlier my mom had been visiting our new house in Ohio, and she asked to see our laundry room.

"Now you have a yard big enough to hang your jeans up, but I guess you don't do that. You put them in the dryer," she had said. I winced. I laughed to cover up how uncomfortable I felt being identified as "the one who puts her jeans in the dryer."

Jason did most of our laundry. He knew I didn't like the collecting, the sorting, the changing of loads, the folding, the putting away. It was because it all reminded me of the weekends as a kid, when I felt that housework and chores superseded anything fun. Or maybe it was the overwhelming feeling I got when faced with a pile of clothes, dirty or clean. He washed our clothes, our sheets, our towels. He was adamant about getting out spots: big, small, almost nonexistent, chocolate, blood, coffee, bacon grease, dirt. He made the piles disappear each week as I napped to make the anxiety-induced fatigue disappear.

It didn't matter to me that we put our jeans in the dryer.

Letting go of the laundry, of the dryer, or the idea of hanging my clothes on a line or a rack (which I had attempted many times in my dorm room or apartments) allowed for *more*. It allowed me to figure out who I was without my mom's habits (ones that sometimes became mine), without her worries about the wrinkles in the jeans or the chance of rain when her clothes were outside. It allowed an expunging of my old anticipations of notes requesting my laundry, a mother waiting up for me to walk in the front door late on a Friday night, the worry that I would get in trouble for allowing an opened Elmer's glue bottle to spill onto my teal carpet and dry into a matted mess. Disappearing was the child I was to my mother. In its place was a new rapport between a young mother leaning on her wiser mother for support. It was a safe place to turn when I miscarried my babies, when I didn't know how to carry on with my life, my work, my uncertain journey toward motherhood. In the gap that grew from the disappearance of the child-mother relationship we once had, I grew into my independence, planning my life with Jason: the family we would make, the home we would have, the pets we would adopt, the cars we would buy. In its place was my mom becoming a grandmother. One who could play with Evelyn and then return to her peaceful, quiet home. One who could excitedly text me days before our visit and ask *what foods does Evelyn like? Goldfish crackers? Chocolate milk? Ice cream?*

...

When Evelyn came inside from the laundry line, she was smiling.

"Now let's play!" she had said.

The previous three losses brought us to my daughter—my curious, adventurous, resilient, silly, fun daughter. Evelyn brought happiness to herself and my mom, and a peace to me.

The things left behind created the white space we needed.

[ARTHROGRYPOSIS] ON THE PLAYGROUND

Things Evelyn wanted to be able to do independently on the playground at the beginning of Summer 2020 but couldn't:

1. Climb the steps.
2. Climb the ladder.
3. Monkey bars.
4. Walk over wood chips.
5. Get up on a swing.
6. Pump her legs on the swing.
7. Climb the rock wall.
8. Climb up the slide (like she saw many other kids do, so it must be the right thing to do)

...

The playground was crawling with kids, climbing up the slides, going down the slides, swinging on the bars, shrieking, hiding, running.

Evelyn looked at me and said, "Come on, Mama, come with me!"

"Can't you just try and go on your own?" I responded. "I bet you could do something."

"No, Mama, I need your help!"

The sun outside of the shaded picnic table area was hot. The air was thick, as if we were wading through a swimming pool. *Swimming would have been a better choice*, I thought, *but that is so much work.*

"What do you want to do?" I asked her.

"I want to climb up the slide like that boy did!"

"Okay," I said, "But you know that slides are for going down, right? And that you have to be able to go up fast in order to not slide back down, right?"

"Yeah, I know."

I watched her get both feet up on the bottom of the slide.

"Help! Help!"

"Evelyn, you can do this. You barely started."

Every trip to a playground made us see what muscles needed more strengthening. Her right shoulder was barely moving, the bone of the joint stretched out the skin. I could see the place where the muscle should have been. The muscle that should cover the bones, stretch over the arm and wrap around to her back. The one that would allow her to lift her arm up to the sky. The one that would allow her to hold her arm stretched outward, as if she were a bird flying. The muscle that would let her do arm circles, swim with a freestyle stroke, swing a baseball bat, hold up a cafeteria tray.

We had begun working on her hip flexors—the muscles that help lift a leg.

"Don't swing your leg around like that, Evelyn. Try and pull it up. Bend your knee," I said to her as she tried to climb the ladder. Her foot swung out making a big half-circle landing arch-down onto the rung. It slipped when she tried to pull her knee up.

"Help! Help!"

"Evelyn, what did I just say about swinging your leg like that? You have to try and pull it up. *Bend your knee*. Like this."

"I know but that's hard."

"If you whine, I'm not going to help you, Evelyn. I can't do the whining."

Her whine droned. High-pitched and putting anxiety where it didn't belong. A foot on the ladder rung could be fixed.

I heard my own exhale, a release of breath that, if I had been doing yoga instead of holding back what I really wanted to say, would have been considered ujjayi pranayama breathing. I would have been calming the mind while warming the body. Instead, it was more like a valve released on a pressure cooker.

She's almost up.
Why can't she make it herself?
How long do I have to do this for?
Why can't she just play like the other kids?

I'm done.

I watched as Evelyn grabbed the top bars and used her arms to pull. They had the strength her legs lacked.

When (if ever) will this be easier?

DIARY REMIX

Sophia,

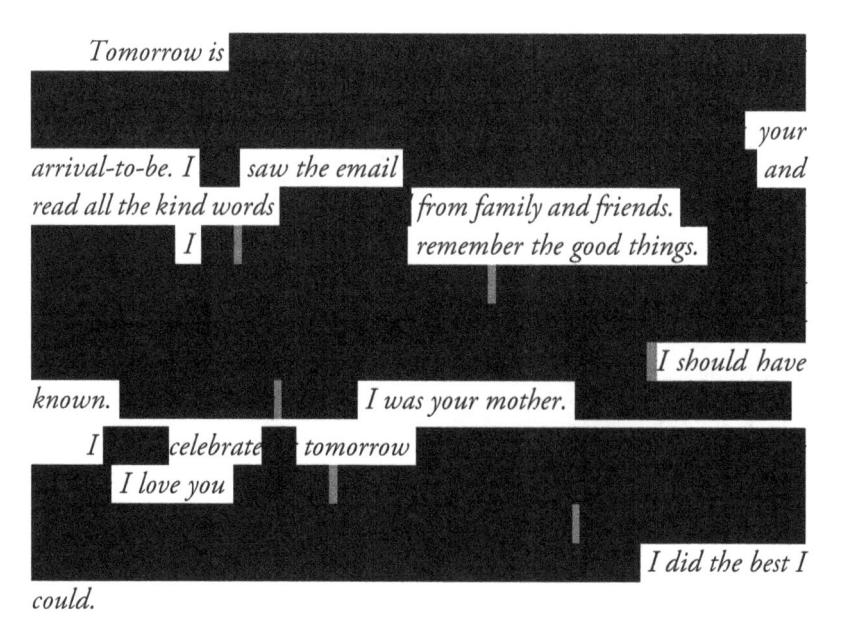

    Tomorrow is arrival-to-be. I saw the email your and read all the kind words from family and friends. I remember the good things. I should have known. I was your mother. I celebrate tomorrow I love you I did the best I could.

    I love you, sweet baby.

LAURA GADDIS

Dear Sophia,

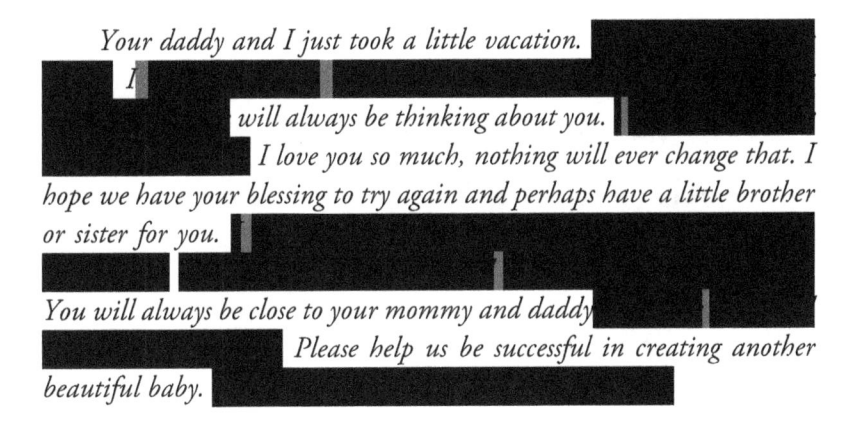

Your daddy and I just took a little vacation. ▮▮▮ *will always be thinking about you.* ▮▮▮ *I love you so much, nothing will ever change that. I hope we have your blessing to try again and perhaps have a little brother or sister for you.* ▮▮▮

You will always be close to your mommy and daddy ▮▮▮ *Please help us be successful in creating another beautiful baby.*

Love you always,
Mommy

CRITERIA I NEED TO MEET TO MANAGE MY GAD (PART 4 OF 4)

Criterion 1: Attend therapy.

Finally listen to Jason, after years of him suggesting this, and find a person who specializes in anxiety and depression, who can listen to you without you having to fear that you're untreatable, and spill your guts to this person. Go once every two weeks (at first), and then when you start to utilize the coping skills (the deep breathing, the meditation, the mindfulness, the thought stopping to slow your brain down) you will go once every three weeks, then once a month. Use these sessions to talk about everything: your worries about your unstable employment as a short-term contracted adjunct instructor, your (perceived) inability to even teach college students, your fear that your daughter Evelyn will never walk, your frustration when you hear your husband struggling to get your two-year-old to put on her clothes, and how to squash your impulse to jump in and fix everything going on in her room. Continue going until you and your therapist decide you've improved enough to do it on your own. She'll suggest it once, in April, six months after you begin seeing her, but you'll continue booking appointments for the next year-and-a-half anyway until your insurance changes to one she doesn't take. By this point, though, you'll feel ready. You'll have learned to self-calm, even if it's a process you do repeatedly over the course of one day, one hour, one minute.

Criterion 2: Take medication.

Take two different pills, because why not? But really, take two because you'll need them. One (the small blue one) will help you with the two-in-the-morning insomnia, the very insomnia that keeps you up until four A.M.—every, single, night. The other (the larger pink one) will calm your daytime running brain, the brain that runs like how new cars now have daytime running lights that you cannot figure out how to turn off, even when you have been instructed to do this by the young girl at the ticket hut who asked you to turn off your headlights while driving through the Christmas lights for the enjoyment of everyone! Check the "anxiety" box off with your primary care doctor the summer after you start therapy (even if you aren't sure that you've been officially diagnosed with "generalized anxiety disorder" by your therapist because you never see her notes and only see the diagnosis when the online pharmacy fills the order). The doctor's nurse will take a cheek swab and send your DNA for testing to see which antidepressant drugs should work the best with your makeup. You may never have heard of such a test before, but it exists. The test may be able to predict which pills will increase your serotonin levels appropriately, but it won't predict which will give you debilitating headaches. Allow your doctor to walk you through a series of medications that will first cause your idiopathic intracranial hypertension (random extra brain fluid that just won't drain and causes pressure headaches) to run amok, your brain ballooning into the empty space in your skull so hard you fear the bone may crack. The large pink pill that your doctor will finally prescribe won't do that, though. Don't give up.

Criterion 3: Live mindfully.

Like really do this, don't just say you are now a mindful person. When you are walking your pug, Rocky, up and down the street, watch the birds that soar overhead and flap their gray and white wings as they land on a tree branch, one that toggles as they come to stillness. What kinds of birds are there? Robins, and blue jays, and even a pileated woodpecker. Get a bird app on your phone so you can learn each name, keep track of each one that lands in your yard. Watch the robins use the nest on the porch light right outside your kitchen window. The mother robin sits in the nest for days—over two weeks, in fact—and you wonder what she thinks about. How mindful she must be in order to sit and do nothing. Or rather, you watch her doing everything to make sure her baby robins are born.

Criterion 4: Meditate daily (or almost daily).

Download the "Calm" app on your phone and use the free trial until you are convinced that meditation is actually working. At first, it feels trite. You listen to "Tamara," the woman who writes and narrates many of the sessions. You will do all of the introduction sessions, followed by the anxiety and the relationship ones. After a year, you will try to do meditation every night before bed to help your daytime running brain calm down (to assist the little blue pills, of course.) You can sit, cross-legged, under the covers of your bed, back snuggled up against the three pillows you stack along the headboard. Use your air pods so you don't bother Jason who is reading a book, or scrolling through Reddit on his phone, or playing Super Mario Bros. on the Nintendo Switch, next to you in bed. Hit play on your phone's screen, turn your phone over so the lighted screen won't shine through your lids, and close your eyes. Hands rest half on your kneecaps, half on your thighs. The breathing begins. Ujjayi breath, as in the pranayama (or breathing control) you practice in yoga every morning. The audible inhale will trail up the back of your throat, the constriction causing a wave sound. The exhale sounds the same. Same tightened throat, slow release. Sit for the ten (or so) minutes, and on nights that you feel like you need an extra session, do another.

THINGS I...

...didn't think Evelyn could do:

1. Live, breathe, and survive on her own with no wires, isolettes, monitors, feeding tubes, and oxygen cannulas.
2. Maintain a body temperature warm enough to be allowed to sleep in a crib.
3. Drink from a bottle.
4. Eat solid food without her gag reflex throwing it back up and onto my hand.
5. Crawl on hands and knees (not army crawl).
6. Stand up holding onto furniture
7. Walk, take steps (independent of a walker).
8. Take more steps than just three.
9. Take more steps than just twelve.
10. Walk herself around the house at her own free will.
11. Stand up from the floor without holding onto a couch, or a coffee table, or my hand.
12. Pick up a toy she dropped on the floor and stand up.
13. Throw a ball underhand.
14. Throw a ball overhand.
15. Use two hands to throw the ball.
16. Put on a shirt.
17. Put on pants.
18. Put on socks.
19. Put on her shoes.

20. Put on her coat, zip her coat, put on a hood.
21. Run with her friends in a game of duck-duck-goose.
22. Jump in a fresh rain puddle on the sidewalk outside of her daycare.
23. Climb the stairs to her bedroom, to the basement, to anywhere.
24. Climb into her car seat.
25. Buckle her car seat.
26. Climb out of the car seat (and get out of the car).
27. Walk up and down a curb.
28. Walk on grass (especially long, uncut grass).
29. Walk on wood chips to the playground.
30. Be as happy as a child could possibly be.

...have realized Evelyn *can* do[24]

1. All of the above (most notably number 30) except 21 and 22.

...expect Evelyn *will* do[25]

1. All of the above.

---

[24] A list constantly in motion, one that feels stagnant for months before shifting dramatically. Her first physical therapist from North Caroline, Denise, told me before we moved to Ohio: *there is nothing this girl won't do. She's just on her own timeline.*

[25] A list that's just a constant.

YOU ARE MY SUNSHINE

Evelyn and I rocked on the glider every day. I was still on maternity leave, staying with her until she was at least six months old before sending her to daycare. With her birth two months before we expected, we had little purchased ahead of time: no more than a crib, mattress, and a car seat. We had some clothes and diapers from the baby shower the month prior, but no one had given us preemie sizes. We had planned to buy a glider—the right of passage for new parents with dreams of feeding their babies, rocking their babies, and singing to their babies in comfort—but didn't think we'd need it yet.

Amazon will deliver a CHAIR? I had asked Jason when he suggested we have it delivered to our third-floor apartment. *Sure! You can get anything from Amazon,* he said. From Evelyn's bedside in the NICU, we put the oversized, overstuffed chair into our virtual shopping cart. It arrived in two days and awaited Evelyn's arrival four weeks later.

Her four-pound body laid on my legs. I watched her take the bottle. Her mouth opened slightly, her eyes stayed closed, like a fish blindly searching for the flakes that float from the top of the water. The nipple of the bottle disappeared between her slender lips, and we rocked.

She had found her suck reflex before she was discharged from the hospital—a requirement for her departure. The goal at first was small: a few milliliters of milk. Then ten, then twenty, then twenty-five, and eventually the full bottle of thirty. The first night she took thirty, Jason and I had already gone home for the day. When we returned in the morning, a nurse had left the empty bottle on Evelyn's isolette bed with a note saying *I drank the whole bottle!*

The nurses had given us extra bottles and nipples as a parting gift to use until Evelyn graduated to the Dr. Brown's bottles we had bought from Target.

At home, her feeding schedule and my pumping schedule worked in tandem: I fed, she ate, I pumped, she slept. I labelled the milk bag with the current date and the date three months out. One bag went into the freezer, and I took out another to thaw.

"Okay, baby, I have to put you down so I can pump," I told her.

She laid in her rocker with vibrations that were supposed to soothe her. I pulled her back-and-forth a few times, until I was confident she seemed peaceful. I sat on the bed, only a few feet away from her, and began assembling the pumping equipment. The tubes on the machine. The funnels that attached the tubes to my body. The bottles to the ends of the funnels.

Evelyn watched.

I hooked up the nursing bra, the kind outfitted with two holes for the flanges to go through and from where the bottles hung. I turned the dial. The whirring began.

Evelyn began crying.

"Don't cry, Evie," I said.

She didn't stop.

"Mommy's right here."

She wailed. High-pitched, arching notes that reverberated her vocal cords and my fused, vertebrae-less spine.

Jason was at his office at Wake Forest University. The neighbors to the left of us and across the breezeway were strangers. My co-workers were busy at the psychology clinic twenty minutes away. My parents, who lived in Wisconsin, had gone home from their visit.

Jason's mother was back in Virginia. His aunt and grandmother had not yet made it out from Maryland.

Evelyn and I were alone.

I couldn't stop the machine. My breasts were engorged; it couldn't wait, not if I wanted to prevent a third round of mastitis[26]. The cords kept me bound to the mechanical plastic evil necessity.

I couldn't get to Evelyn.

"Please stop crying, baby…"

Her tones took on a curvature that bent them up to the top of a scale; to the shrillest of keys on the right end of a keyboard, and back down. It reminded me of when I was young and took piano lessons. The trill, the fast flickering between two notes, my fingers flying as fast as they could go.

I remembered a commercial for Johnson & Johnson baby wash with a mother gently singing "You Are My Sunshine" as she sat on the edge of the bathtub. I recognized the melody, the cheeriness it exuded. But I had never learned the lyrics. I pulled out my phone and searched.

Once I found them, I sang:

You are my sunshine, my only sunshine,
You make me happy when skies are gray…

---

[26] Painful lines of red crossed my chest, the clogged milk ducts preventing the milk from being expressed. The fluid that was so vital to Evelyn's growth had nowhere to go. Neither did the pain. The first time I had mastitis, I thought I had the flu: chills, fever, body aches. Jason called the doctor, who mercifully did not ask me to be seen before prescribing the antibiotics. The second time I had it, the ache in my ankle bones gave it away. I pumped through the infection, the pulling of my skin feeling like a ripping of flesh. I said *if I get this one more time, I'm done with pumping*. A month later, I packed up my pump for good.

My voice was dampened by tears, the grinding gears, Evelyn's rhythmic wails.

You'll never know, dear,
How much I love you,
Please don't take my sunshine away.

I held my phone in my left hand, my right clutched the half-filled bottles. If they fell, which they hadn't yet, but if they did, I would have just one more reason to cry.

The other night, dear,
As I lay sleeping,
I dreamt I held you by my side.
When I awoke dear,
I was mistaken.
So I hung my head and I cried.

"It's okay, baby. Evelyn…. Evelyn…look at Mommy! Look here baby! You're okay. I'm almost done. You're okay. I'm okay. We're okay."

You are my sunshine,
My only sunshine.
You make me happy,
When skies are gray.

It was a little too soon to shut down the machine, but it was close enough. The bottles filled quicker than they had during the first days, days when mere droplets lined the inside of the bottle, what the NICU nurses said *would give your baby the taste at least and we'll supplement with donated milk.* It was time to turn the dial on the pump's speed down. The grinding softened to a hum.

You'll never know, dear,
How much I'll love you.
Please don't take my sunshine away.

Evelyn quieted. Her screams turned to whimpers, and then faded into saliva-filled gurgles.

"I'm almost done, baby. Then we can snuggle."

Her face was wet. The tears, the spit, the mucus running from her nostrils, the agony I didn't understand.

Was she hungry? If only I could have gotten the breastfeeding to work, for her to understand to latch onto my nipple instead of the bottle, but after five weeks of exclusively using bottles in the NICU, she just didn't understand how much simpler this whole process could have been for us both.

I'll always love you,
And make you happy.
And I know you'll say the same.
But if you leave me,
To love another,
You'll regret it all one day.

My voice softened on these last words as we finally lingered in a silent room.

...

I later learned that "You Are My Sunshine" became popularized in 1940 by Jimmie Davis, a former college professor, criminal court clerk, and hillbilly singer. He later became the governor of Louisiana, and the song became the second state song, behind "Give Me Louisiana." Davis sang "You Are My Sunshine" at his campaign rallies. It became a symbol for what is American, the simple melody easy to learn, the lyrics of the chorus uplifting. When I read the verses, especially the lines most left out *(but if you leave me, I dreamt I held you by my side, but I was mistaken, you'll regret it all one day)* I thought of how we were told we'd lose Evelyn just like my other babies, how she wouldn't survive two holes in her heart, how she was born too early and had to prove her strength and will to live. She was my sunshine. Please don't take her away, too.

I heard others sing the song, most recently Johnny Cash's solemn version on YouTube when I was searching for lyrics. Many have sung the haunting words, each putting their own take on what they mean, how the melody flowed (fast and jazzy, slow and weepy): Louis Armstrong, Gene Autry, Sandi Jensen and Salli Flynn backed by the Lawrence Welk Orchestra, Bing Crosby, Norman Blake on the "O Brother Where Art Thou" soundtrack... the teachers in Moore, Oklahoma to their fifteen young students as they hid in the bathrooms while they waited for the tornadoes to blow past, mothers bathing newborns and lulling them to sleep, me with a crying newborn, not yet five pounds, grasping for something to soothe us both.

...

One early July night when Evelyn was four years old, on the brink of turning five, I was putting her to bed. She brushed her teeth (then I took a turn to reach the molars), she used the potty (then I helped her wipe and straighten out her bunched-up underwear), she came into her bedroom, I asked *did you wash your hands?* she responded *yes….,* she returned to the bathroom and I heard the water run, and she came to the bed where I sat.

"Hi, baby. Thanks for *actually* washing. Remember germs, right?"

"Yucky!" she said.

"Okay, so what book do you want to read?"

"*Kindergarten Here I Come!*" she said.

It was a new book she had received for her birthday. It was one I had read to her the past two nights.

"Okay, but after tonight, we'll take a break from it."

When she wasn't tired, when her muscles still had enough life in them to get her legs onto the metal bedframe and her biceps could still pull on the covers, she could get herself onto the mattress. But tonight, like most nights, her limbs were loose, her efforts coming out in grunts. Her hands grasped at the bedding. She swung her legs to the left, trying to catch a foot on the edge of the mattress. Each time, though, she slipped down just enough to keep her from getting up.

I pulled her onto the bed.

"Ugh, baby, you're getting to be so big," I said. Her thirty-five-pound body stretched my arms, pulled at my knuckles, and popped my wrist as I lifted her up and swung her so her feet landed by me. "Let's get your night shoes on."

Since she was a baby, we had been treating her club feet. First in the NICU with tiny white casts that covered her foot-to-knee. One morning we came back to find nurses had written *'Hope'* and *'Love'* on with purple and blue markers.

When she came home, we visited a pediatric orthopedic doctor. We sat in the exam room, Evelyn sitting on my lap, my purse under the chair. When I was not much older than her, I sat with *my* dad waiting for the orthopedic doctor to examine my spine, my ribs, my deformities. To learn if progress was made, or if my scoliosis had worsened. I wondered how much of this Evelyn would remember when *she* was thirty-five.

At Evelyn's first appointment, we learned the casting that she had in the NICU was the wrong kind.

"That's the Kite method," Dr. Ravish had explained. "I do the Ponseti method. It's the most widely used method of casting for treating clubfoot. The 'gold standard.'"

When he told us we'd have to let her feet be cast-free for three weeks to let them return to the clubbed positions, I was angry at the NICU doctor for having taken us on the wrong path. *Why didn't the NICU guy know better?* I asked Jason on the ride home. *He's a doctor, right?*[27]

We learned how to undo the mistake:

Step 1: Full-leg casts—ones that now covered her feet and stretched up to her hips. Change every week for eight weeks.

1.1: Load Evelyn into her car seat after finding pants that will cover her heavy, cast legs; keep her calm during the thirty-minute drive to and from Dr. Ravish's office. Repeat every Friday.

---

[27] I searched the internet for the NICU doctor and found he worked in a clinic that primarily treated adult patients. *Why the hell do they let him treat babies in the NICU?!* I wondered.

1.2: Watch the casting assistant start up his drill. Listen to the loud grinding, watch the blade spinning close to Evelyn's leg.

1.3: Hold Evelyn's hands to keep her lying back. Keep her still. Watch her face for signs of fear, of crying, of confusion. Say: *It's okay, baby. You're doing so good, baby. Almost done!* while holding in my own tears and desire to grab her from the table and safely wrap her back up in the stroller.

1.4: Help Evelyn sit up as the cast assistant wets the fiberglass—a wrap in a color I picked (the only choice I had in this matter). Watch Dr. Ravish hold Evelyn's left foot at a ninety-degree angle, knee bent.

1.5: Keep Evelyn still so the cast assistant can wrap the gauze, the pink or blue or purple or red soggy strip around and around and around until it is thick and heavier than Evelyn's whole body. Repeat on the right leg.

Step 2 (after the first eight weeks): Get Evelyn fitted for the Ponseti braces (our 'night shoes').

Each day: Put foot in, make sure heel is down in the bottom of the shoe, buckle three times (middle buckle *always* first).

2.1: Pull buckles so tight it feels like her metatarsal bones might fracture.

> **Pro Tip:** When you think you've tightened it enough, go for one hole tighter. Have her wear shoes for twenty-three hours a day for the first year (one hour allowed for bathing).

Step 3: After one year of diligence, wear the Ponseti braces for twelve hours a day.

Step 4: Maintain for the next four years.

Step 5: Wean off of Ponseti braces to five nights a week.

5.1: Celebrate "no shoes nights" by putting fuzzy red socks on Evelyn's liberated feet.

Step 6: ?

...

Evelyn always cooperated with the shoes. By the time she was four-almost-five, she didn't know a night without them.

"But I *HAVE* to sleep with them on!" she said.

"Dr. Chandran said your feet will be okay," Jason said.

"If we notice anything changing, we'll let Dr. Chandran know right away," I added.

"We have to tell her right away!" Evelyn said, emphasizing each word with a wave of her index finger.

When we had our first no-shoes night, we commemorated with a family snuggle—Jason on one side, me on the other—in her bed, for reassurance.

We left her alone to sleep, her feet free to rub within her red fuzzy socks and the soft flowered sheets. I, too, always rubbed my bare feet on the soft sheets to help me go to sleep.

The Ponseti shoes challenged me every time it was my turn to put them on Evelyn.

"Toes up," I said.

Her right toes naturally angled outward up to ninety degrees from the center. It made her foot look as if it were attached sideways. Sometimes when she stopped walking, she'd stand so her right toes pointed behind her. *It's a rotation of the bone starting from the knee,* her orthopedic doctor in Ohio, Dr. Chandran, told us. *Asking her to rotate it straight would be awkward for her, just like it I asked you to turn your arm and hold it there.* Yet, Evelyn could do it easily when asked, no pain, no crying.

"Don't forget the tissue!" she said.

The tissue, folded into a small square, protected the top of her ankle from the buckles rubbing. The tissue was our design. The "Pringle" chip came with the shoe. Attached to the middle leather strap it was supposed to be the protector. It just wasn't enough.

"Got it, baby."

I pulled the middle strap over the tissue, over the chip, and into the metal clasp. The strap stretched as I tugged it hard. The first time I had to strap her newborn foot into the shoe, I was certain I would break her. Having clubfoot made her feet smaller than normal. She wore six-month shoes when she was two-years old.

Now, I yanked. Each hole that I could stretch out of the strap reminded me of her arch collapsing back onto itself, her toes reaching once again toward each other, her stubby digits with toenails curved and scrunched. We witnessed the curvature happen once when Dr. Ravish requested we start the casting over. It wasn't something I ever wanted to see again. Jason and I were in charge of these shoes. We were the ones protecting her feet.

I clicked the metal bar to the sole of one shoe, then to the other. The metal bar tethered her feet together

"Okay, baby, get comfy."

Evelyn wiggled up the mattress until her head reached her squishy hedgehog pillow. Her feet dragged behind.

"Let's sing one song. What do you want to hear?" I asked.

"The stake song."

"*Which* one?"

"The stake song!"

I thought for a moment. I pictured a steak. We never ate steak.

I mentally perused the brief catalogue of songs I knew by heart. Memorizing lyrics was a weakness of mine. Unless it was a song that I loved—the melody, the beat, the invitation to dance, the minor key it's in, the dramatic tone, the beauty in the words—lyrics expired in my memory. My mom used to sing *Inch worm, inch worm, measuring the marigolds...* but never *You Are My Sunshine*.

Sometimes songs reminded me of a meaningful time, like Christmas at the ranch house I grew up in, or old country music that played in my parents' kitchen, and in the garage, and on the car radio, and in my dad's basement workshop. Often singing "do do do" or "hmm mmm" to cover for the words I didn't know, or just finding replacement words altogether, there were few songs I sang enough times that I could actually memorize.[28]

"Oh, you mean the *mistake* song?"

"Yeah!" she waved her arms at me in exasperation, her weakened right shoulder not allowing her arm to extend as high as the left. Yet, both of her hands waved at me as if she were saying *get with it, Mom!*

"Okay, but you have to sing with me."

She nodded.

You are my sunshine,
My only sunshine.

Her soprano voice squeaked over my alto tone.

You make me happy,
When skies are gray.

---

[28] *Song lyrics I know accurately by heart:* Most Garth Brooks songs (I had been obsessed with him since I was eight), Islands in the Stream, a duet by Kenny Rogers and Dolly Parton (even this has become shaky in my adulthood), Twinkle-Twinkle Little Star, Jingle Bells, and You Are my Sunshine.
Song lyrics I cannot remember or have to make up: everything else.

MOSAIC

Her words came a beat after mine. She was trying to match the lyrics, remember them, and filling in with mumbles when necessary.

You'll never know, dear,
How much I love you.
Please don't take my sunshine away.

I inhaled enough to carry me through the next verse. She smiled and waited.

The other night, dear,
As I lay sleeping,
I dreamt I held you by my side.
When I awoke, dear,
I was **mistaken***.*
So I hung my head and I cried.

"Wait!" said Evelyn. She held her hand up in my face.
"What?" I said.
"Did you look for me in my room?"
"Well, no, I guess not."
"You need to look for me in my room! I'm always right here!"
"Okay, baby, next time I will do that." I laughed. "Let's keep going."

You are my sunshine,
My only sunshine.
You make me happy,

When skies are gray.

You'll never know dear,

How much I love you,

(Evelyn pointed her right index finger at me when she yelled "you")

Please don't take my sunshine away.

We paused. I looked at her. Her eyes seemed to beg me to continue.

I'll always love you,

And make you happy,

And I hope you'll say the same.

But if you leave me,

To love another,

You'll regret it all one day.

"But I'm not going anywhere, Mama. I'm right here!"

"That's good, baby," I said. I leaned in and wrapped my arms around her.

"And what does 'one day' mean?" she asked.

"Just like...sometime in the future."

"I'll always be here, Mama."

"I hope so, baby," I said. I sat up. "We have one more verse. Ready?"

You are my sunshine,

My only sunshine.

You make me happy,

MOSAIC

When skies are gray.
You'll never know dear,
How much I love you,
Please don't take my sunshine away.

Evelyn yawned, her mouth stretching into a long misshapen 'O.' We had a picture of her from the NICU with her mouth in the same shape, a photo from a professional photographer working for Capturing Hopes, a volunteer organization that gave families free pictures of their treasured babies. In this moment, like so many others, was a snapshot of what we had.

Her arm wrapped around Larry, her rainbow llama.

"Goodnight, Evelyn. You sleep *so so so* good so we can have a lot of fun tomorrow, okay?"

Her fingers traced my cheek, my nose, my eyelids.

"Don't poke me in the eye, Ev!" I said. The tingling on my cheek and nose lingered. I soaked in the warmth from her finger, the softness of her skin.

"You sleep good, too, Mommy. You need your energy!" She had learned that the advice I always gave her was good for me, too.

"You're right. I definitely do."

I hit the orange button on her owl night-light. The white glow faded as the owl aged each year. The button on her tiger night-light required four pushes, bypassing the white glow, the green, and the blue, until it shined purple—her favorite color. I reached behind her basket of stuffed animals sitting upon her bookshelf to grasp the off switch to her reading lamp.

"Night-night, Evelyn. See you in the morning."

The laminated paper *EVELYN* hung from her doorknob swayed and I pulled it away from the jamb so it wouldn't get caught.

"Night-night, Mama."

I shut the door and walked away. Away from the buckles and the leather straps, away from the shoes and the metal bar, away from the owl nightlight and the tiger one, away from my Evelyn so she could rest her tired body tonight.

I shut the door on my previous pregnancy losses, on the realization that I'd never carry another healthy child, on the sadness that stings my soul every time a friend says *I'm pregnant! We're having another one! We wanted Sammy to have a sibling!*, on the confusion and wonder about when (or if) my body could do what a woman's body should or meet the expectation that is there, on the casts and braces and night shoes, on the hours spent on physical therapy and the crunchies and leg lifts and snow angels and arm raises done at home between the appointments. On the boisterous, too-smart-for-her-age toddler who was softly falling asleep under the butterflies on her comforter.

I shut the door on the fear of not having a child of my own, of losing another one, of fearing for my child's life.

I shut the door on regrets, worries, anxieties, darkened days.

I shut the door knowing we would start all over again, tomorrow.

CRY AND MTF ON

Evelyn was four and wanted to try dance lessons. The other parents sitting with me easily slipped on their daughters' ballet shoes. I held Evelyn steady with my right arm while my left tried to pry the end of the fake pink leather over the end of her plastic ankle-foot-orthotics. My index finger pinched between the hardened plastic that held her foot in place and the shoe that made her feel like a ballerina.

She had asked to do dance class after her preschool teachers taught her how to "nod, shake, move your hips" from Blazer Fresh's hit kid tune "Banana, Banana, Meatball." Kid hip-hop was hardly her first exposure to dancing, but I was delighted when she asked to "be a ballerina."

...

Once, I was cooking dinner with her, a soup in my new Ninja Foodi pressure cooker, and I danced around the island counter to get to the refrigerator.

"Don't do that!" Evelyn said.

"Why not?"

"Because!"

"It's not nice to tell people to not dance if they want to," I told her. "Do you want to dance with me?"

I can remember dancing when I was her age, often at random times. One time I put white mittens on my feet and danced out of my bedroom into the living room where my mom and dad sat. *Look at me!* I said. When they laughed, my anxieties about everything—making friends at school, our house burning down at night, someone breaking in, being kidnapped as I walked home from school—disappeared.

Despite my irrational fears in life, I always danced and sang. Or it's because of my irrational fears that I did these things. It was something about myself that I always liked.

"C'mon," I said to Evelyn. "Let's dance."

I went over to the stool where she sat and I held her hands. She slid off the seat, and as her feet hit the ground, we both paused. Her legs wavered, the right more than the left. That knee was still weaker and bent inward. *Valgus* her orthotics maker and physical therapist called it.

It's also called knocked knees, they told us at every appointment, as if we would forget from month to month, or just needed the layman's term to understand.

Evelyn's knees touched every time she stood from a chair; she couldn't stand up with space between them. Valgus is a tibiofemoral angle (or the anatomy of the shin and thigh bones meeting at the knee) that measures greater than ten degrees. Evelyn's right foot turned outward when walking, up to ninety degrees if we didn't remind her to use *monkey foot* (a term Evelyn came up with on her own as recommended by her physical therapist, Ms. Nicole) to remember to walk with her foot at forty-five degrees. Forty-five degrees was not normal. It's not the angle my own foot points when I ambulate. But it would be *good enough* for a child whose tibia rotates outward from below her knee.

"Whoa," she said.

"I got you," I said. "You ready?"

Evelyn nodded, saying *no* then *yes* in the way she often did. Her brain needed time to vocalize thoughts before landing on the right one. Or it could be that she liked to try and trick me. Either way, I knew it wasn't because her brain had a misshapen part like my high-risk doctor had said all those months ago. Even if her brain parts were more "triangular" than it should have been, it almost seemed to make her wiser.

The song was something by Ed Sheeran. Something with a drumbeat, an acoustic guitar, and lyrics of love and loss.

"Let's do this," I said.

Evelyn hung on to both of my hands as we began to sway. She had difficulty picking up her feet. Her right one shuffled more than the left. Her weakened hip flexor muscles didn't allow her knees to rise the way a marching soldier could. Instead, she alternated her weight from hip-to-hip.

Back and forth. Back and forth.

Right then left. Right then left.

With each shift, her white-sparkle tennis shoes stomped the floor. If the little pieces of glitter weren't glued on so well, shiny shards would have covered our kitchen like snowfall dusting a field.

...

At ballet, with her leather slipper shoes now clinging to the outer edges of her heels, I helped Evelyn stand up. I held her hand as she stepped down the three shallow stairs to the dance floor.

"Let go, Mommy!"

"I'm sorry, Evelyn," I said. "I want to make sure you are safe. That's my job."

She wandered away from me and toward the group of girls who took off running toward Ms. Ashley, their teacher. Evelyn's gait was lopsided, her right foot still dragging more than the left. She often said *watch me run fast, Mama!* when she tried to run, yet she was capable of little more than a shuffle.

She grabbed a mat from the bin and walked it out to the middle of the floor. I wanted to run out there. I wanted to grab the mat. I wanted to spread it out for her, neatly between two other toddlers who had already done so and were lying flat giggling. I wanted to tell the other parents to stop staring—because I was *sure* they were staring—at the girl who walked with yellow braces and whose right knee buckled in.

I watched carefully, calling out *are you all right?* when her toe grazed an uneven surface and made her fall. She started to stand without responding. Her legs slowly pushed her back up. She tipped forward and caught herself with her hands on the floor. The second time she pushed up, she made it all the way.

I turned away. I knew she needed to do this for herself. I knew that the older she got, the less she would want my help. The other parents were talking. Some wandered out into the hallway.

I distracted myself: a text message, a Facebook post, an email. The new featured items at Aldi for the week.

I wondered if doing this made me less of a mother, or more of one.

When I looked back up, Evelyn had her mat out. She had found her place between Ms. Ashley and a little blond-haired girl. Her legs out long; her body folded in half. Her flexibility amazed me. For all her constricted joints and muscle tightening, she could touch her toes as easily as I could clasp my hands.

The girls got up from their stretches. Most ran back to the bin, throwing their mats in. Evelyn stayed on the floor. She started on the short end of the mat and rolled it. Each flip of the mat turned it into a beautifully cared for piece of equipment. She tried to stand. One hand on her mat, the other on the floor, her feet tried to get beneath her. Her butt up in the air as if she were doing a yoga pose. She scooted her feet forward. I assumed the deep lunge in her knees burned her thighs as doing chair pose always burned mine. Her right foot pointed outward. Her right knee skewed inward.

I held my breath...

She pushed up...

C'mon, baby, I thought. (Or was that out loud?)

Her right leg gave out. Her foot slipped from beneath her.

She was no longer doing a down dog yoga position. She was just down.

"Aw, man," I said.

I closed my eyes. For a moment it was dark. The sorrow came in like disappointment when the protagonist dies at the end of a play. My eyes dampened.

But then the houselights came on. The curtain reopened. I saw Evelyn out there, standing. Carrying her mat. Smiling. Waving at me.

I stopped the impending cry. Barely. Sometimes it doesn't work that way. Sometimes, I hide in my bedroom and shut the door. I cover my face in my hands and let tears wash over my palms. The cleanse feels good. It feels bad. I often wonder, *how can I cry so much when Evelyn doesn't?*

Dance class carried on. Ms. Ashley had the girls line up. In front of them was a mirrored wall.

"And plié!" Ms. Ashley said. "Do this, girls! Girls! Look here. Like this!"

The line disintegrated. Girls started twirling (not a plié) or running (also not a plié).

"Girls!"

Evelyn held Ms. Ashley's hand. She steadied her balance. Her feet already naturally turned outward. Her muscles long, lean, flexible. She bent her knees.

A plié.

When ballet class was over, Evelyn walked back to me. She had gotten her hand stamps from Ms. Ashley, the sign of a class gone by. A dance completed. Now she was ready to put on her tennis shoes and MTF on.

The ballet shoes fought coming off as much as they did going on. I felt the skin on my finger stretch as I won the battle with the elastic band that had attached itself to her Velcro.

Evelyn kept smiling.

She was excited to talk about the scarves they twirled and the stuffed monkeys they threw into the air.

"Did you see me, Mommy?"

"Of course I did, baby."

"Did I do good?"

"You did! I saw you twirl and chassé and plié."

"I fell a lot."

"It's okay, baby. You know what I liked?"

Evelyn shrugged. Her right shoulder, the one with little muscle tone covering her bones, didn't make it as high as the left.

"I liked that every time you fell, you got right back up. That's what you need to do."

We put our coats on. She held my hand in the parking lot.

"No cars coming!" Evelyn said.

"Then let's go!"

We Moved The Fuck On.

Part 4

THINGS I HAVE LEARNED

Learning: the acquisition of knowledge or skills through experience, study, or by being taught.

I don't know everything. I wish I did. I wish I knew how to let my past-self know that future-self would be okay. Future-self would actually turn out better than okay. Future-self would have a smart, funny, spirited child who struggles with gross motor delay (but who doesn't struggle with something?). Future-self would leave one career to explore another one—one with less certainty about income and success. Future-self would be living in a home that is warmed in the winter, cooled in the warm Miami Valley summers, and filled with so much laughter the whole neighborhood swells with sounds of *hahaha*! every day. Future-self would become present-self, who is a mother, a wife, a daughter, a human finding happiness.

Motherhood: 1. the state of being a mother; maternity, 2. the qualities or spirit of a mother, 3. mothers collectively.

It's complicated how I could love like a mother, dream about my future child like a mother, postulate what color will be her favorite, what foods she will eat and to which she will say 'yuck,' what color hair, eyes, skin (freckled or not) she will have. Yet, I knew that when the doctors told us that something was wrong with our first baby, that she wouldn't survive long past birth (if she even made it that far), I never felt more like a mother.

My mother was a mother when she pulled me aside in the kitchen at Jason's and my home two weeks before Christmas—a few days after we learned the terrible news—and told me, "You have to make the choice that's best for you. The baby matters, but you are my baby and you matter, too. We have to take care of you."

She was a mother when she hugged my still-pregnant body and then resumed helping me finish cooking the chicken marsala stew I had chosen to make for a pre-holiday family meal.

She was a mother when she collected the dishes off of the makeshift dining room table we had set up in the living room of our cozy ranch.

She was a mother when she sat with me on the green corduroy couch, her arm around my shoulders, as we smiled for a photo.

She was a mother when she came to the hospital the day I was admitted due to bleeding, and when she tried to keep my mind on things less dire than my going into early labor by reading to me the hospital lunch menu.

She was a mother when she and my father, returning the day Sophia was born, agreed to see Sophia's deceased body, and was led away by the nurse who offered to take my parents there.

Moving Forward: 1. To advance in position or progress: The player moved forward and kicked the ball toward the net. 'We've had some setbacks, but it's important that we keep moving forward with our original schedule in mind.' 2. To cause or compel someone or something to advance in position or progress.

I was driving home from work one day a few years after Sophia's death. I was just newly pregnant with Evelyn. It was a typical North Carolina February day—chillier than I would have believed a southern state to be. The tie of my long winter coat still fit around my midsection. NPR was on the radio. The show "Fresh Air" came on every afternoon between four and five when I was on my way home. The interviewer was talking to Kenneth Lonergan, the writer and director of "Manchester by the Sea." They talked about the movie's premise, a man who is left to raise his recently deceased brother's child. I felt tears welling up. Ever since Sophia, I couldn't help but cry at others' loss--even those that are fictitious or imagined.

"Moving on is different than moving forward," Lonergan had said.

I thought about those words the rest of my drive home. I had heard his explanation, how he wasn't advocating for just letting go of some emotion to make room for the new. Moving on means you forget, but moving forward means you let go of what happened without forgetting the change you sustained from it.

Acceptance: acceptance in human psychology is a person's assent to the reality of a situation, recognizing a process or condition without attempting to change it or protest it.

Please respond with one or more checkmarks in the appropriate box(es):

When did you first accept that Sophia would (and did) die?

Option A: When the doctor first told you she had abnormalities, something like Down Syndrome? (That seemed too breathable, too common, too prevalent, too survivable.)

Option B: When the ultrasound technician at the high-risk appointment couldn't get Sophia to move so she could take the proper measurements, so she had you walk the halls, drink soda, and use the bathroom in the hopes Sophia would roll?

(I didn't feel Sophia move much until the end of her short pregnancy anyway.)

Option C: When the high-risk doctor and genetic counselor told you Sophia wouldn't survive?

(I cried. My thigh muscles shook. My head felt light, as if helium had been pumped into my body. But did I believe it?)

Option D: When she was born?

Option E: When you watched her perish in Jason's hands, when the nurse did her regular heartbeat check and said I have to get the on-call doctor, when the on-call doctor came with his stethoscope (one so large it filled her entire chest) and listened motionlessly, when he pulled the earpieces out and said I'm sorry, she's gone? (But she was just breathing! She breathed longer than the medical staff said she would! She might breathe again if I just hold her again? Put her to my warm chest, cover her body with the striped hospital blanket? Put her back in my womb where she began?)

Option F: When you arrived at the funeral home and the funeral director told you the process for cremation: Her body will be placed in a metal box to catch the ashes…

(**Extra option**—check here if appropriate) Or when he led you to the urn room and told you to choose the model we wanted?

Option G: When you began blogging about her, writing about your grief, sharing your work, and receiving messages stating: we lost our baby, too, I wish I could write about my son the way you write about your daughter, thank you for sharing your story?

Option H: When you were finally a family of three: Jason, Evelyn, and you?

Option I: When you explained to Evelyn that she has an older sister, she lives on top of Mommy and Daddy's dresser, and showed her the small silver heart engraved with Sophia Grace Gaddis 12-31-10?

Duality of Emotion: feeling more than one emotion at a time, even if they seem to be opposing each other.

The day after Sophia was born, my sister came to visit me at the hospital. Sarah brought along a Tupperware filled with curried chicken salad and rolls. She declined seeing her niece's body, a choice I understood was difficult for her at the time. I wondered if she felt so much love that it brought equal amounts of pain to even think about witnessing the body.

Six months later, I hosted Sarah's baby shower in our backyard. I didn't know at the time she visited me in the hospital that she was pregnant with her first child. When she told me, I said *congratulations!* and then hung up the phone and cried. But I loved Sarah so much, my only sibling (only eleven months twenty-six days older than me), one of the only people I could say I knew my whole life, who always was there to play with, to share a car with when we both got our licenses, to be the person whom I went to when I was mad at our parents. I knew I was the one who had to give her a baby shower.

I handmade sugar cookies in the shape of owls, frosted each one, and added chocolate eyes. I ordered catered sandwiches and supplemented with bruschetta and orange sherbet mimosas (for the non-pregnant guests). I glued colored pieces of paper and images of flowers onto a poster board in order to walk around and ask guests *do you want to play a guessing game?* I made gift bags for guests, put out decorations of plastic baby rattles, and bottles, and tiny bits of *ItsAGirl!* confetti.

I got up in front of the guests, assembled on lawn chairs on our patio, our driveway, and spilling onto the grass in order to welcome them and thank them for their generosity and kindness in celebration of Sarah and Andy's baby.

    During a brief moment, I stepped into the house and into our living room. For the first time since the party started, I was alone. I looked out the picture window, the cars lining the streets for Sarah, for her husband, for their baby. I wiped away a tear. I took a deep breath and rejoined the party.

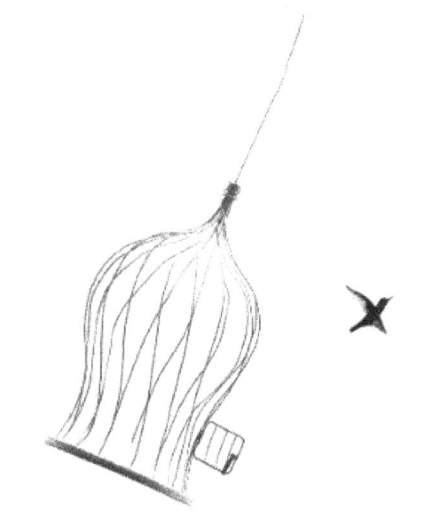

NOTES

MAKING IT
Norton, Amy. "Couples' Risk of Break-Up after Pregnancy Loss." *Reuters*. April 8, 2010. www.reuters.com/article/us-couples-loss/couples-risk-of-break-up-higher-after-pregnancy-loss-idUSTRE6374DU20100408

GENERALIZED ANXIETY DISORDER (GAD)
American Psychiatric Association. Diagnostic and Statistical Manual of Mental Disorders, 5th, ed. American Psychiatric Publishing, 2013.

THE ODDS
Ferry, Dave. "Everything You Know About Surviving Rip Currents is Wrong." *Outdoors Online*. June 22, 2016.
www.outsideonline.com/2089696/everything-you-know-about-surviving-rip-currents-wrong

Miceli, Courtney. "Spider silk is five times stronger than steel--now, scientists know why." *Science Magazine*. November 20, 2018.
www.sciencemag.org/news/2018/11/spider-silk-five-times-stronger-steel-now-scientists-know-why

WALKING THE RIVER OF GRIEF
"What does Buddhism teach about life after death?" *BBC*.
www.bbc.co.uk/bitesize/guides/zfts4wx/revision/3

ALL THE THINGS
MTHFR Mutation, *Lab Tests Online*, labtestsonline.org/tests/mthfr-mutation

WELL-MEANING PEOPLE
Adriaens, I. ,Smitz, J., Jacquet, P. "The current knowledge on radiosensitivity of ovarian follicle development stages." *Human Reproductive Update*. Vol. 15 Issue 3. January 16, 2009, https://academic.oup.com/humupd/article/15/3/359/747352

Yvonne Butler Tobah, M.D., "Pregnancy Week by Week." *Mayo Clinic*. www.mayoclinic.org/healthy-lifestyle/pregnancy-week-by-week/expert-answers/x-ray-during-pregnancy/faq-20058264, retrieved 11/21/19.

FUSION
Hyde, Beverly. "An Interview Study of Pregnant Women's Attitudes to Ultrasound Scanning." *Social Science Medicine*, Pergamon Press Ltd. Vol. 22, No. 5, 1986, pp 587-92.

YOU ARE MY SUNSHINE
Deusner, Stephen. "'You Are My Sunshine': How a maudlin song became a children's classic." *Salon*. May 26, 2013, www.salon.com/2013/05/26/you_are_my_sunshine_how_a_maudlin_song_became_a_childrens_classic/

ACKNOWLEDGEMENTS

When I lost my first baby, Sophia, my husband encouraged me to go back to writing—a love I had since childhood but one that had long been put on the back burner in favor of a career in psychology. That tiny suggestion to start a blog was the seed that sprouted, grew, and has spread like dandelions in a field of brilliant yellow. It became my writing journey. I am forever grateful to Jason for not only giving me this idea, but for his constant support and encouragement through all the years that followed—from encouraging me when my writing was rejected (many, many times), to celebrating my wins of finally getting publications, getting accepted into and finishing my MFA program, and especially for when Mosaic found its home with Unsolicited Press. We have weathered a lot together and I am proud to have him as my partner in all I do.

My children are my greatest inspiration. It is as much a wonder in this world to watch a tiny baby be born and perish within a night as it is to watch another child thrive and discover the world one iota at a time. As I entered the role of motherhood, I was not prepared for how to take in all that came my way, but I am forever grateful for every minute. Sophia helped me find my way back to writing, and my daughter, Evelyn, keeps my writing going.

My best writing is not done in solitary, and for that I cannot express enough gratitude to all the exceptional mentors, writers, and peers whom I have worked with. Firstly, I am deeply indebted to those at Miami University who believed in Mosaic from the beginning and who have helped it take form along the way. Deepest gratitude to Dr. TaraShea Nesbit for her gentle guidance and encouragement from the moment this book was born. Thank you to Dr. Jody Bates and Professor Brian Roley for graciously spending time with my work and offering ways to make it the best it could be. Professor Margaret Luongo added suggestions during my last workshop experience in the MFA, and it was her insight that that helped me finish my thesis.Thank you to all of my peers and classmates during the MFA years who gave generous critique: Rachel Giesel Grimm, Maddy Krob, Brianna Verdugo-Chow, Frenci Nguyen, Jen Sammons, Kelsey Timmerman, Lloyd Mullens, Dalanie Beach, Sof Voet, Harrison Chinekotam Mmerenu, Chiamaka Onu-Okpara, K Anand-Gall, and Theresa Skrzat, Sam Gutelle, Louisa Pavlik, Matt Boyarsky. These are the people who read many pieces of Mosaic and helped it take the form that you see it in today. It was an invaluable two years filled with workshopping, editing, and humbling gratitude.

I'm also indebted to those wiser, established writers who have gifted me with knowledge before and after graduate school. Thank you to Kiese Laymon and Ann Hood for their brilliant insights into writing memoir. They helped shape me into a great storyteller.

Thank you to my family: my parents, my sister, my grandma, and my extended family for always believing in my writing. I send extra gratitude to my mother, who I see so much of myself in. Without having her in my life, I would not be who I am today.

Thank you to my amazing publisher, Unsolicited Press. Memoir is not an easy genre to bring into the published world, and you saw the vision I had and the story I had to tell in the way I wanted to tell it. It is a dream come true to have my book out in the hands of readers. Thank you to Summer for careful edits of my work and for supporting a year of women authors.

Finally, thank you to my readers, starting way back to the inception of my blog in 2011. Some of you I know well, some are acquaintances, and others strangers. I keep writing because all of your voices joined the conversation.

It is with gratitude that the following essays have been previously published:

"Erasure," Evening Street Review, Forthcoming 2022

"Fusion," The Stonecoast Review, Issue 16, January 2022

"Things They Don't Teach You," 805 Lit+Art Magazine, December 2021

"Cry and MTF On," The Dillydoun Review, Issue 9, October 2021

"Well-Meaning People," Ligeia Magazine, Summer 2021. *Nominated for a 2021 Pushcart Prize*

"You Are My Sunshine," Adelaide Literary Magazine, May 2021

"I Knew," "Hoosier," and "Journey", The Avalon Literary Review, April 2021

ABOUT THE AUTHOR

Laura Gaddis is a writer, book coach, and educator living in Oxford, Ohio. With a former career in clinical psychology, and more recently earning her MFA in creative writing from the Miami University (of Ohio), she is interested in writing about the human condition, whether it be her own or that of others. Laura writes fiction and nonfiction that centers around the idea that through storytelling we can connect humanity on profound levels, elevating us to be better for ourselves and for each other. Her writing has been nominated for a Pushcart Prize and she has publications in literary nonfiction, poetry, and humor fiction in *Thin Air Magazine, The Avalon Literary Review, Adelaide Literary Magazine, Ligeia Magazine, Pif Magazine, Vita Brevis Press, Kitchen Sink Magazine, The Dillydoun Review, Evening Street Review, 805 Lit + Art, Stonecoast Review, The Weekly Humorist.* Additionally, she has published articles on parenting and mental health on the popular websites Scary Mommy, Tiny Buddha, and The Mighty. Laura resides in Oxford, OH with her husband, daughter, and pug Rocky.

ABOUT THE PRESS

Unsolicited Press is based out of Portland, Oregon and focuses on the works of the unsung and underrepresented. As a womxn-owned, all-volunteer small publisher that doesn't worry about profits as much as championing exceptional literature, we have the privilege of partnering with authors skirting the fringes of the lit world. We've worked with emerging and award-winning authors such as Amy Shimshon-Santo, Brook Bhagat, Elisa Carlsen, Tara Stillions Whitehead, and Anne Leigh Parrish.

Learn more at unsolicitedpress.com. Find us on Instagram, X, Facebook, Pinterest, Bsky, Threads, YouTube, and LinkedIn. Unsolicited Press also writes a snarky newsletter on Substack.